The Quality Advantage

A Strategic Guide for Health Care Leaders

Julianne M. Morath

Foreword by
Paul Batalden, MD

press

Health *info*Source
An American Hospital Association Company
Chicago

Printed in the United States of America—12/98

Cover design by Amy Aves

Library of Congress Cataloging-in-Publication Data

Morath, Julianne M.
   The quality advantage : a strategic guide for health care leaders / by Julianne M. Morath.
         p.   cm.
      Includes bibliographical references and index.
      ISBN 1-55648-256-6
      1. Medical care—Quality control.   2. Total quality management.
I. Title.
      [DNLM: 1. Quality Assurance, Health Care—organization & administration.   2. Total Quality Management—organization & administration.   3. Health Services Administration—organization & administration. 4. Organizational Innovation. W 84.1M831q 1998]
RA399.A1M67 1998
362.1′068′5—dc21
DNLM/DLC
for Library of Congress   98–36020
                                                                                    CIP

Item number: 169411

About the Authors

Julianne M. Morath, MS, RN, is system vice president for quality, education, and performance effectiveness for Allina Health System, Minnetonka, MN. She also has administrative responsibility for the oncology program at Abbott Northwestern Hospital and is a member of the executive staff. Ms. Morath has 23 years of experience as a patient care executive. She holds academic appointments at the University of Cincinnati, Brown University, and the University of Minnesota, among others. She has done extensive postgraduate work in organizational leadership. Ms. Morath is a frequent speaker on systems thinking, patient care delivery design, and topics related to quality and organizational learning.

Joachim Roski, PhD, MPH, serves as director in the Quality and Performance Effectiveness Division of Allina Health System, Minneapolis, MN. He directs the development and implementation of a comprehensive performance and clinical quality measurement and improvement system. Dr. Roski is also one of Allina Health System's key contributors in the area of developing and testing innovative population health improvement approaches by bridging intervention approaches rooted in a medical or public health model. He serves as principal investigator and co-investigator on a number of research projects related to health care quality improvement, care system innovation, and population health improvement. He is a frequent presenter at conferences and is well published in these areas. Dr. Roski holds faculty appointments at the University of Minnesota and St. Thomas University, St. Paul.

This effort is dedicated to Dr. Gilbert Maienknecht, father, mentor, and reliable compass.

Contents

Foreword

Health care leaders and their organizations are being asked today to change and improve the quality and value of their care. What will health care organizations and their leaders need to be able to do to thrive in the time immediately ahead? They will need the capacity to do the following:

- Improve patient and customer service
- Redesign the care for patients

Improving the service for patients and other customers involves setting the priority, developing knowledge of the preferences of patients, mapping the points of connection between the system and the people who depend on it, measuring and monitoring the performance of the work done in those "connections," and using that information to change and improve the relevant processes.

The capacity to redesign the care for patients involves the capacity to improve the outcomes of care, the ability to improve value by taking out work and cost year after year, and the capacity to increase pride and joy in work and learning for health professionals while doing this redesign work. Knowing about the best anywhere can fuel local learning in a supportive environment.

Although many seem to agree with these needs for the future, few have acted to require incumbents or candidates for positions of leadership to demonstrate their personal skill in leading the change and improvement of health care. Why?

Morath has offered a very practical description of the approach that she and her colleagues at Allina have used to design and initially operate a system-wide process for the improvement of the quality and value of health care. The book is written by and for thoughtful leaders and practitioners. The work of leaders is described with helpful examples from health care and from other service settings. Helpful questions abound. The author and her colleagues recognize the need to focus on what matters in improving patient care. She knows and offers others insight into the importance of designing human resource and employee development systems that promote an environment supportive of the changes needed in health care.

Measuring and monitoring the improvement of the main work of health care professionals and their organizations—providing health care—is still in its infancy. We are much better at counting the volumes of work or financial status of what is done. The authors tell the story of Allina's journey to modify their measurement system to help them monitor their main work.

Knowing what to do is different than doing it. The authors offer insight into their efforts to get started. Their reflection on their actions offers the reader insight into the thinking and design of those actions.

Those interested in selecting and developing leaders of health care for the future could use this account to frame their own question as they establish the suitability of candidates and programs for the important work of leading the establishment of cultures that promote and improve the quality and value of health care.

Paul Batalden, MD
Center for the Evaluative Clinical Sciences
Dartmouth Medical School

Preface

This book focuses on issues and applications for quality as a business strategy. The working definition of quality for this book is that *quality* means meeting or exceeding customer requirements. Using the focus on the customer, Kano described quality as the degree to which the work and the need or requirement of the customer correspond.[1] He used three categories of focus: defect reduction, waste reduction, and innovation.

1. *Defect reduction:* A defect is anti-need. A defect can hurt, delay, or produce an incorrect action. Error, or more accurately stated, medical accident, is defect. When accidents occur, harm is done when good was intended. In considering the basics of providing a safe environment in which care is received and provided, the focus is on reducing defects or accidents. This is done through meticulous attention in developing a culture of quality through a foundation of safety and using the science available to understand work processes and human strengths and capabilities to predict and prevent accidents.

2. *Waste reduction:* Waste occurs when energy is used up, but nothing is produced that brings value or satisfies the need of the customer. Waste is costly. Eliminating waste and efficiently and effectively meeting customer need are the focus of improvement. This includes eliminating waste in all its forms—excess materials, time, duplication, unintended variation, lack of focused or aligned action.

3. *Innovation:* Innovation occurs when a new need is discovered and met. It requires knowledge of customers and insight into their preferences. Innovation requires a culture that is constantly learning, improving, and seeking to anticipate and create the future. In considering innovation, the focus is on the ability to partner with customers, to use the energy of the company toward creating positive change, and

to avoid dissipating talent and energy through failures to lead, implement, and consistently advance strategy.

There is so much work in all of these areas in health care that it is the job of leaders to focus on the priorities.

LEADERSHIP STRATEGIES FOR BUILDING A CULTURE OF QUALITY

J. M. Juran, founder and chairman emeritus of the Juran Institute, who was decorated by the emperor of Japan for "the development of quality control in Japan and the facilitation of United States and Japanese friendship," was author of many books on the subject of quality. In his book *Juran on Leadership for Quality: An Executive Handbook,*[2] he outlined critical questions for senior managers.

- What role does quality play in the success of my company?
- How can I evaluate my company's status in respect to quality?
- How shall we, as a company, manage for quality in the face of new challenges?
- What must we, as a company, do that is different from what we have been doing?
- What road shall we follow to go from where we are to where we want to be?
- What should I, as a manager, do that is different from what I have been doing?

His book systematically addresses the answers to these questions. The most helpful concept in building the model for quality is the Juran Trilogy: managing for quality is accomplished through the management of quality planning, quality control, and quality improvement. Table 1 summarizes these processes.[3]

Whereas Juran offers managerial action steps toward establishing an approach to quality, W. Edward Deming offers 14 leadership principles of quality.[4] Dr. Deming, a leader in the quality movement, said leaders must do the following:

1. Create consistency of purpose for the improvement of products and services.
2. Adopt the new philosophy.

TABLE 1. The Juran Trilogy: Managing for Quality

Quality Planning	Quality Control	Quality Improvement
Determine who the customers are	Evaluate actual product performance	Establish the infrastructure
Determine the needs of the customers	Compare actual performance to produce goals	Identify the improvement projects
Develop product features that respond to customers' needs	Act on the difference	Establish project teams
Develop processes to produce the product features		Provide the teams with resources, training, and motivation to diagnose the causes, stimulate remedies, and establish controls to hold the gains
Transfer the plans to the operating forces		

Reprinted with the permission of The Free Press, a Division of Simon & Schuster from *Juran on Leadership for Quality: An Executive Handbook,* by J. M. Juran. Copyright © 1989 by Juran Institute, Inc.

3. Cease the dependence on mass inspection.
4. End the practice of awarding business on price tag alone.
5. Improve constantly and forever the system of production and service.
6. Institute training and retraining.
7. Institute leadership.
8. Drive out fear.
9. Break down barriers between staff areas.
10. Eliminate slogans, exhortations, and targets for the workforce.
11. Eliminate numerical quotas.
12. Remove barriers to pride of workmanship.
13. Institute a rigorous program of education and retraining.
14. Take actions to accomplish the transformation.

Developing ways in which the principles can be brought to life within the organization is the work of leadership. This book addresses specific leadership strategies for building a culture of quality through which these principles can be brought to life in the work of the organization.

Quality Requires Commitment

Creating a quality business culture is important work. It underscores what is important to people. If quality is part of the organizational fabric, the organizational practices will exceed the needs of customers, protect professional ethics, and provide the safety necessary for employees to question, explore, and improve work.

It is, therefore, not to be entered into lightly. Some people have described the start of a total quality journey as being like dancing with a bear—you don't walk away before the dance is over. It requires commitment, constancy of purpose, and endurance because the dance is continuous. Stated in organizational terms, William O'Brien, retired CEO of Hanover Insurance Companies, is quoted as saying: "I talk with people all over the country about learning (total quality) organizations, and the response is always very positive. If this type of organization is so widely preferred, why don't people create such organizations? I think the answer is leadership. People have no real comprehension of the type of commitment it requires to build such an organization."[5]

Peter Senge, senior lecturer at the Massachusetts Institute of Technology and a cutting-edge thinker about organizations and quality, talks about this leadership issue in the following way: "Our traditional view of leaders—as special people who set the direction, make the key decisions, and energize the troops—is deeply rooted in an individualistic and nonsystemic world view. Especially in the West, leaders are heroes—great men (and occasionally women) who rise to the fore in times of crisis. So long as such myths prevail, they reinforce a focus on short-term events and charismatic heroes rather than on systemic forces and collective learning."[6]

The commitment and skill necessary to focus on information, systemic forces, and collective learning are the cornerstones of quality and the embodiment of Dr. Deming's 14 principles.

Quality Requires a Willingness to Change

Just as quality has transformed American business, the leader's crucial role in promoting quality as a successful business strategy will transform the ongoing responsibilities, the interpersonal relationships, even the daily personal habits of leaders in the organizations that pursue this strategy. For those leaders whose organizations have begun the quality journey—and certainly for those leaders who have taken it upon themselves to be the inspirational leaders of that journey in their organizations—there needs to be a substantive transformation in their approach to leadership. They must put aside their traditional views of leadership and acquire new and essential skills. Fortunately, there are dozens of examples—successes and failures—that can help today's leaders develop the talent and commitment necessary to bring quality to their organizations in meaningful ways.

For quality to be the driving force in health care strategy, the leaders in health care organizations must first recognize and commit to quality as a business imperative. Then, having done so, the leaders must understand what this means in tangible terms to them personally. The emphasis here is on tangible terms: *What does a commitment to quality mean in strategy, communication, and action?* This is not an abstract notion; leading an industry in quality is a contact sport.

Until the leader figures this out, there will be a gap between senior management's intention and the front line staff's experience. This book raises the question of how leaders can change the culture of their organizations and begin to exercise their leadership within an organization so that status quo and inaction are not acceptable. Leaders who are serious about making a commitment to quality need to answer two challenging questions before they take action:

1. Do you care about quality?
2. What are you going to do about it?

STRUCTURE OF THIS BOOK

This book is divided into 11 chapters. Chapter 1 describes actions that leaders can take to make quality a priority within their organizations. These include creating a learning environment and appropriate systems, defining new roles and responsibilities for managers at all levels, and incorporating quality in their personal beliefs and behavior. Chapter 2 encourages creation of a clinician-customer partnership and describes various models that are part of what is known as the total quality evolution. It also offers a framework that can be used to facilitate the partnering process. Chapter 3 focuses on quality as a business imperative by offering ways to look at error reduction and increase safety. To underscore leadership's role in this, the chapter provides lessons learned from other industries. Chapter 4 presents three models for building a practical model for quality: the broad organizational model, the value chain model, and the care delivery process model. Chapter 5 focuses on creating the infrastructure an organization needs to pursue its quality goal. This includes offering development and training opportunities, choosing the right team sponsors and facilitators, and implementing quality assessment methods. Chapter 6 describes how to recognize the conditions within an organization that make it ready for change and improvement and uses a case study to illustrate how to harness and direct the creative energy needed to make change happen. Chapter 7 hones in on getting started on the road toward improvement. It discusses the criteria to consider when selecting clinical areas of focus and the process involved in making a selection as well as in selecting appropriate measurement methods. Chapter 8 uses the quality measurement system developed at Allina Health System (AHS) to illustrate how an organization can build in a system for measuring performance, improvement, and innovation methods. Chapter 9 focuses on the characteristics of organizations committed to quality and discusses the needs and responsibilities of various stakeholders within the organization with regard to performance improvement measures. Chapter 10 offers a real-life application of the concepts discussed in this book. Using the experience at AHS, it describes the actual steps that one organization took to launch its quality strategy. Finally, chapter 11 looks at organizational quality improvement as an opportunity for those who work in health care to instill pride, joy, and meaning into what they do and to return to the fundamental elements that define the soul of the health care organization.

References

1. Lillrank, P., and N. Kano, "Quality Control Circles in Japanese Industry," *Continuous Improvement,* no. 19 (1989): 294.

2. Juran, J. M., *Juran on Leadership for Quality: An Executive Handbook,* The Juran Institute, Inc. (New York: The Free Press, 1989).

3. Juran, pp. 20–1.

4. Horak, B., *Strategic Planning in Healthcare—Building a Quality-Based Plan Step by Step* (New York: Quality Resources, Kause Organization, Ltd., 1997): 4.

5. O'Brien, W. In Senge, P., "The Leader's New Work," *Sloan Management Review* 32, no. 1 (Fall, 1990): 14.

6. Senge, P., "The Leader's New Work," *Sloan Management Review* 32, no. 1 (Fall, 1990): 14.

Acknowledgments

What is the right care? What is important to customers about their health care? What do health professionals need to know about continually improving care? These questions have launched us toward a new and challenging frontier in understanding quality in health care. I have the privilege of working with distinguished leaders who, by their very actions, are creating answers to these questions.

I would like to acknowledge several of these leaders who have been pivotal in advancing my learning and practice and who model the way for others in their focus and insistence in unsurpassed quality.

Thank you to Gordon M. Sprenger, Executive Officer of Allina Health System, Minneapolis, Minnesota; Paul Batalden, MD, Health Care Improvement Leadership Development Center for Evaluative Clinical Services, Dartmouth-Hitchcock Medical Center, Hanover, New Hampshire; James Ehlen, MD, President of Allina Health System; Joyce Clifford, RN, PhD, Vice President of Nursing and Nurse-in-Chief, Beth Israel-Deaconess Health System, Boston, Massachusetts; Marie Manthey, RN, MSN, President, Creative Nursing Management, Minneapolis, Minnesota; and Robert K. Spinner, System Vice President and President, Allina Hospitals, Allina Health System.

I would also like to thank the friends, colleagues, and patients whom I have had the privilege to work, serve, and learn with. They have helped shape the content of this book. I specifically want to acknowledge the commitment, talent, and generosity of employees, medical staff, and board members of Allina who continually strive to improve patient and customer service and redesign care to achieve results of unsurpassed quality.

I would also like to acknowledge the following contributors for their efforts in producing this book:

Joachim Roski, PhD, MPH, Program Director, Clinical Measurement in the division of Quality, Education and Performance Effectiveness for the Allina Health System in Minneapolis, Minnesota.

Dr. Roski co-authored chapter 8, Building an Integrated Quality Measurement and Improvement System, with Julianne Morath. He is the author of chapter 7, Selecting a Focus and Getting Started, and chapter 9, Using Measurement for Performance Management. Dr. Roski leads the design of pilot studies to test innovations in health improvement and care delivery and works with interdisciplinary teams to design clinical measurement systems. His work on smoking cessation has received national recognition.

Robert Jeddeloh, MD, authored the case study for improving asthma care contained in chapter 6, Making Change Happen. Dr. Jeddeloh is Director of Care System Innovation and Associate Medical Director for Public Programs for Allina Health System. Dr. Jeddeloh has received national recognition for his work in tobacco control and smoking cessation, school-based care, and comprehensive strategies for the care of children with asthma. He is an expert resource in improvement strategies for emergency, community, and clinic-based care.

The Crackleberry Group, based in Woodbury, Minnesota, provided research assistance in the examination of the Baldrige quality award winning organizations.

Nancy Garner Ebert provided ongoing encouragement, writing advice, and editorial expertise in this project. Ms. Ebert is a marketing communications specialist for Allina Health System, Minneapolis, Minnesota.

Coral Sampson provided expert technical and logistical support in the manuscript preparation. She stepped into the process and restored its energy through her untiring commitment to see the project through. Ms. Sampson works with the School of Nursing at the University of Minnesota.

Thank you also to Michelle Fredrickson, who coordinated the production of the figures displayed in the chapters and who was helpful in cross-checking references contained in this document. Ms. Fredrickson is executive secretary to Julianne Morath.

Thank you to Janice Ophoven, MD, and Bryan Bushick, MD, who participated as members of the quality team and architects in the early development of an integrated approach to quality in Allina.

1

Defining Leadership's Roles and Responsibilities

Quality will not have the strategic importance it should within an organization until the board of directors and the CEO of the health care organization are explicit about quality as a business imperative. The first question this statement raises is whether the board of directors and CEO are convinced that quality is an imperative. Do leaders believe the study of small area variation and capacity, led by the work of Dr. John Wennberg and colleagues?[1] Do leaders believe the studies of medical errors and the costs of preventable errors? Evidence brought forward by Dr. Lucian Leape suggests that there are more than 100,000 preventable deaths and more than $8.6 billion in costs related to adverse events in American hospitals each year.[2] Studies conducted at the SEI Center for Advanced Studies in Management at Wharton describe the actions of companies that will survive in the next century: delivering what the customer wants in product and experience, encouraging employees to make decisions and have meaning in their work, learning and acting quickly, and creating value for all its constituents.[3] Is your health care organization prepared? Most important, society—our patients and members—are telling us we must do things better and safer and in greater partnership than we have done before.[4] With this evidence, leadership has the responsibility to make its intentions concerning quality explicit and visible and to lead the organization toward this goal.

This chapter describes the actions that leaders can take to make quality a strategic priority within their organizations.

ASK THE RIGHT QUESTIONS

Asking the right questions and holding people accountable for finding the answers may be the most valuable role of leaders in

1

building a quality culture. The leader's role is to embed and expand quality in the organization. People pay attention to the leader. The questions that the leader asks help focus the company. Leaders should ask questions not only to gather information but also to stimulate responses and find ways to do business cheaper, faster, and better.[5] In this way, leaders require that improvement take place. Leaders who are skilled in asking difficult questions and who are prepared to hear the answers are those who drive change improve performance and competitiveness and improve themselves as leaders. The questions they ask might include the following: Why do we do it this way? Is there a better way? What would it cost? What do our competitors do that is different and better? What could we do—should we do—to become better in this area? These questions encourage taking action rather than just gathering information. Similarly, leaders can use questions to develop a management style that fosters the development of and contributions from employees. For example, the question, "What can I do to help you be more effective in your contributions to quality improvement?" is a question that will move employees and the organization forward.

A good example of how this can be applied may be found in the Henry Ford Health Care System. The staff members of this system are distinguished by their pursuit of key questions about what matters in their service to customers and the performance of the organization. The questions are formalized and answered through their measurement system of key performance indicators. In this system, the CEO and the board chairperson consistently ask the following questions: What is best-in-class in this area? What is our experience? What are we doing toward improvement? The answers to these questions identify what needs to be done to improve the work. They focus the attention of the organization. Questions expose what is valued, monitored, and rewarded within an organization. Through questions, the leader makes clear the organization's values and priorities and creates an environment that encourages a well-informed, prepared workforce ready to search for best practice.

CREATE A NEW ENVIRONMENT

Before exploring the specific leadership roles necessary to build a culture of quality, a general discussion of the leaders' new responsibilities in quality may be helpful. In his article "The Leader's New Work: Building Learning Organizations,"[6] Senge focuses the role of leadership on creating institutions that are oriented toward learning, rather than toward controlling, and toward cultivating one's natural curiosity and ability to continually improve, rather than performing for others. He quotes Dr. Deming, who said, "Our prevailing system of management has destroyed our people." He goes on to say: "People are born with intrinsic motivation, self-esteem, dignity, curiosity to learn, joy in learning. The forces of destruction begin with toddlers—a prize for the best Halloween costume, grades in school, gold stars, and on up through the university. On the job, people, teams, divisions are ranked—reward for the one at the top, punishment at the bottom. MBO, quotas, incentive pay, business plans, put together separately, division by division, cause further loss, unknown and unknowable."[7] Senge says corporations create the very conditions that predestine them to mediocre performance by focusing on performing for someone else's approval—the CEO, the board of directors, the shareholders.[8]

In reality, superior performance is achieved through knowledge of the customer and an environment that encourages learning, which is why the questions leaders ask are so critical. These questions create the environment of inquiry and learning. Senge gives us an historical view: "The old days when a Henry Ford, Alfred Sloan or Tom Watson learned for the organization are gone. In an increasingly dynamic, interdependent and unpredictable world, it is simply no longer possible for anyone to 'figure it all out at the top.' The old model, 'the top thinks and the local acts,' must now give way to integrating thinking and acting at all levels. While the challenge is great, so is the potential payoff."[9]

Former Citibank CEO Walter Wriston said, "The person who figures out how to harness the collective genius of the people in his or her organization is going to blow the competition away."[10] This is the power of quality as a business strategy.

In his work, Senge explores the leader's responsibility for learning: "Leadership in learning organizations centers on subtler and ultimately more important work. In a learning organization, leaders' roles differ dramatically from that of the charismatic decision maker. Leaders are designers, teachers, and stewards. These roles require new skills: the ability to build shared vision, to bring to the surface and challenge prevailing mental models, and to foster more systemic patterns of thinking. In short, leaders in learning organizations are responsible for building organizations where people are continually expanding their capabilities to shape their future—that is, leaders are responsible for learning."[11]

Quality and improvement are based on two fundamental principles: learning and creating a system.

Learning

Creating the environment of learning and striving for unsurpassed quality are crucial. Leaders are instrumental in creating the culture that enables people to tell the truth and allows the development of processes through which those in the organization can learn from the experience.

There is a legendary story of developing leadership at IBM. An IBM executive lost an account. It produced a loss of $2 million to the company, a loss that was expected to be recovered by that same executive in new business. A day after the loss, the executive was called into the CEO's office. The CEO told the executive that he had followed his career and his work, then presented the executive with a new business opportunity to assemble a team, develop the strategies, and lead the implementation of a new international business venture. As the executive was leaving the CEO's office, he told the CEO how excited he was about the opportunity and how he had thought that he had been called into the office to be fired. The CEO responded: "Fire you? Why would I fire you after just spending $2 million training you?"[12]

This example illustrates the power of leadership in nurturing employees through their mistakes. It is part of the cost of developing leaders and creating an environment of safety, learning, and improvement.

Creating a System

W. Edwards Deming referred to improvement knowledge as "a system for profound knowledge."[13] It consists of four domains: knowledge of a system, knowledge of variation, knowledge of psychology, and the theory of knowledge.

Knowledge of a system is a powerful construct. Dr. Paul Batalden says that for leaders to understand the work of the organization as a system and lead and manage for improvement, they must be able to answer three questions: How do we make what we make? Why do we make what we make? How do we improve what we make?[14]

These are deceptively simple questions. Batalden said that answering these questions leads to an understanding of the organization as a system and the work of improvement.[15] Pursuing answers to the first question (How do we make what we make?) requires learning about what is actually produced in terms of products or services. Answering this question precisely begins to identify key processes of the organization and leads to understanding of the current state. The second question (Why do we make what we make?) requires understanding the connection between what the organization does and the needs and desires of the customer and market. It begins to explore value-points of the market and to make judgments about what the organization should be focused on. The third question (How do we improve what we make?) leads toward understanding work from a process flow perspective and the organization as a system. When the organization is structured and understood as a health care system from a process flow perspective, meaningful improvement can be pursued.

ASSESS AND REDEFINE ROLES AND RESPONSIBILITIES

For guidance and direction in how to develop leaders so that they can build a culture of quality, we must look at their roles and responsibilities. The roles range from board member, CEO, and senior manager to middle manager and quality professional.

Board Members

The board is ultimately responsible for the work of the organization and the quality of that work. Specifically, it is responsible for the following:

- Ensuring that improvement is occurring
- Requiring constancy of purpose in the quality journey
- Holding senior leaders accountable for results
- Ensuring that community needs are met
- Leading celebrations of the gains that have been made
- Improving its own methods as a board

Case Illustration: Florida Power and Light   The quality story of Florida Power and Light provides some key lessons for board attention. In the quest for quality, Florida Power and Light aggressively pursued and won the W. Edwards Deming Award for quality control in 1989, which is conferred by the union of Japanese Scientists and Engineers and is a prestigious business award in Japan. Florida Power and Light was the first non-Japanese firm to win this award. However, the utility did so at some cost. Specifically, they spent $400,000 in direct expenses, including the cost of completing an extensive application process, and $885,000 for consultants to prepare them for the award inspectors.[16-19]

Florida Power and Light's aggressive pursuit of quality and customer satisfaction was grounded in the belief that these two factors alone could determine the company's success. As a result, other strategies, such as marketing, were discontinued or de-emphasized. An 85-member quality department was established, and in six months all employees were required to master the Deming method. The statistical control process was made the mandatory problem-solving method. Seventeen hundred teams were formed and tied up in rigid procedures to solve all problems. Supervisors were burdened by overwhelming paperwork, excessive reporting, and declining productivity. To fulfill the Deming Award requirements, a functional review team was required to document and analyze 800 different procedures, right down to how to answer a complaint letter. Supervisors were buried in complex performance indicator tracking. One source reported that it took seven separate steps and a team to identify the steps necessary to move a water cooler.[20]

In retrospect, James L. Broadhead, board chairman and CEO, acknowledged that the zealous program was too much. In a letter to employees in 1990, Broadhead dismantled the quality bureaucracy and what many employees felt was an overemphasis on process and improvement technology for its own sake, a process that interfered with their ability to act and directly serve customers.[21] The 41 indicators were reduced to 3, a focus on the customer and supervisory skills were added to training, and managers were encouraged to fit the process to the issue. Today, Florida Power and Light has a six-member quality department.[22]

Lessons Learned   The postmortem done on the quality story at Florida Power and Light reveals the following lessons for board members. For quality efforts to be meaningful, board members must be able to do the following:

- Understand the business reason for quality: Why are we spending money on this initiative?
- Understand the leaders' work in quality: Why should we commit time and attention to this topic?
- Understand which questions to ask: What questions will help identify what needs to be understood and improved?
- Make sure the right measures are being used: Are the measures creating energy for improvement in critical areas of performance?

- Make sure feedback is going back to the front line for improvement: Are the measures relevant and useful for people to improve their work?
- See results coming back: Are we getting better in ways that matter to our customers?
- Celebrate the gains being made and recognize the work being accomplished: Are we recognizing the results of efforts being made?
- Work on improving the board's work and understanding the process of quality: Are we applying improvements to the work of the board itself?
- Keep public accountability and regulatory compliance as the core responsibility: Are we meeting our obligations to customers to provide safe and effective care?

Board members need to ensure that the processes and systems necessary for quality are in place and that improvement is occurring. Tools such as key performance indicators need to measure what really matters and ensure that the customer requirements are being met. A key lesson is that quality methods support leadership and decision making in the company—they do not replace them. The old adage that if you have only a hammer everything looks like a nail holds true. Decision-making methods, processes, and measures need to be selected appropriate to the issue being addressed. The board can learn about quality by conducting its own self-assessment to ensure that its processes are being improved and its responsibilities met.

Senior Managers

The role of senior managers is to define the system and focus the priorities of the work to be done. Their obligations and responsibilities include the following:

- Creating, sustaining, and perpetuating a shared vision and values
- Understanding the organization as a health care system
- Ensuring safety systems are in place
- Naming the gaps that must be closed between actual and desired performance
- Nurturing commitment to quality principles and leading by example

- Creating a context for work that supports learning and change
- Providing resources for knowledge and skill development in the areas of innovation and learning
- Establishing accountability for trust and improvement
- Recognizing the gains that have been made
- Holding people accountable for changes that must take place at the front line

Case Illustration: Medtronic, Inc.   To illustrate the role of senior management, look toward Medtronic, Inc., the world's leading medical technology company specializing in implantable and invasive therapies. Headquartered in Minneapolis, Medtronic does business in more that 120 countries, with operations organized into 3 global areas: the Americas, Europe/Middle East/Africa, and Asia/Pacific. More than 12,000 employees around the world are actively engaged in 4 businesses made up of 14 business units and 9 ventures.

William George, president of Medtronic, and all other senior managers can and do cite the mission with passion. It is as follows:

- To contribute to human welfare by the application of biomedical engineering in the research, design, manufacture and sale of instruments or appliances that alleviate pain, restore health and extend life.
- To direct our growth in the areas of biomedical engineering where we display maximum strength and ability; to gather people and facilities that tend to augment these areas; to continuously build on these areas through education and knowledge assimilation; to avoid participation in areas where we cannot make unique and worthy contributions.
- To strive without reserve for the greatest possible reliability and quality in our products; to be the unsurpassed standard of comparison and to be recognized as a company of dedication, honesty, integrity and service.
- To make a fair profit on current operations to meet our obligations, sustain our growth and reach our goals.
- To recognize the personal worth of employees by providing an employment framework that allows personal satisfaction in work accomplished, security, advancement opportunity and a means to share in the company's success.
- To maintain good citizenship as a company.[23]

For George and his senior management staff, there is no audience too large (George is connected by E-mail to thousands of employees around the world) or too small (he has frequent one-on-one conversations with new employees) to talk about the mission and the Medtronic pursuit of unsurpassed quality.

Essential components of Medtronic's operations: From the early days, *customer service* was an essential component of Medtronic's operations. At one time, Earl Bakken, the founder of Medtronic, screwdriver in hand, tended to electrical problems in local operating rooms; Palmer Hermundslie, also a founder, piloted his own airplane for emergency deliveries of the company's pacemakers. This hands-on, person-to-person customer service tradition continues today with a U.S. sales team that has doubled in size during the past 10 years and with hundreds of technical support staff members. Supplementing the face-to-face service are professionals who provide technical assistance 24 hours a day via toll-free telephone lines.

An essential element of service at Medtronic is *customer education*, which includes product training sessions, the sponsorship of major medical and scientific seminars and symposia throughout the world, and professionally accredited workshops. The first Bakken Education Center, located at Medtronic's Fridley, Minnesota, headquarters, symbolizes the company's commitment to education. Dedicated in 1990, the center offers state-of-the-art classrooms, hands-on training areas, sophisticated audiovisual equipment, and other facilities to serve physicians, other health care professionals, and Medtronic's sales and technical support staff. Additional Bakken Education Centers are located in cities throughout the United States and in England, Germany, India, Japan, and the Netherlands. Thousands of physicians and associated medical professionals take part in learning sessions at the centers every year, and many others attend company-sponsored symposia at other locations.

The emphasis of Medtronic's senior management on *product quality* began in the early days when the company's founders hand-assembled products in a garage. Quality assurance in those days often meant a close, eyeball inspection by the entire technical staff. Although the means have changed over the years, the insistence of senior managers on quality has continued with ongoing efforts in world-class manufacturing processes, meticulous product testing, and statistical quality controls.

Medtronic's quality efforts: In 1990, Medtronic began its customer-focused quality (CFQ) process, which incorporated all Medtronic quality strategies, programs, and procedures and expanded them throughout all levels of the organization worldwide. CFQ underscores a total commitment on the part of all Medtronic employees to focus on customers' needs and desires by providing them with unsurpassed quality in Medtronic products, services, and relationships.

Examples of the ongoing quality efforts under the direction of senior management include the following:

- Having sales representatives available 24 hours a day to ensure that customers have the appropriate products and support when needed
- Testing Medtronic mechanical heart valves over a span of more than 1 billion cycles—67 percent more than required by the U.S. Food and Drug Administrations guidelines
- Publishing a detailed product performance report (which is unique in the medical industry) that provides performance data on Medtronic's pacemakers and leads
- Conducting customer satisfaction surveys for the collection and assessment of perceptions and imperatives

These quality efforts are directly linked to the development of the Medtronic culture and the legacy of Earl Bakken, through the stories of unsurpassed quality told by George and other Medtronic leaders.

Each holiday season, Medtronic invites customers—the patients and families who have required care resulting in use of a medical device produced by Medtronic—to meet and speak with Medtronic employees about their health care experience. The mission for Medtronic takes on a personal face and lives for the engineers, scientists, and technical and sales staff who design, produce, and distribute the product. Unsurpassed quality and zero defect take on a human life.

Lessons Learned   The lessons learned for senior managers in examining the Medtronic illustration include the following:

- Inspiring a workforce to achieve unsurpassed quality requires direct contact with people and explicit examples of what is important. This is done by appearances at orientation, E-mail messages, and personal disclosures by the leader of his or her passion about the work. It also means bringing the customer inside to meet with employees so that employees are directly connected to the effects that the product they make has on the lives of the customers.
- Investing in the development of people's skills, both technical skills and team skills, is necessary to achieve organizational goals.
- Setting best-of-class standards and measuring performance against those standards focus the attention and energy of the organization.

- Holding management accountable for achieving quality and financial results makes quality non-negotiable.
- Keeping the customer at the center of decision making ensures attention to the fundamental grounding of quality.
- Celebrating the gains the organization has made publicly reinforces performance and creates an incentive for improvement.
- Taking tough-minded action if the values of the company are violated by anyone employed by the company communicates integrity and commitment to purpose.

Middle Managers

Managers nurture the environment and develop the staff resources to integrate quality principles in the workplace. They also model quality principles in their interactions with staff and customers. Their responsibilities include the following:

- Anchoring the work to the vision and mission of the organization
- Planning for quality improvement
- Creating an environment of trust and accountability for improvement
- Intelligently creating and managing change
- Providing developmental opportunities for staff
- Encouraging participation by staff
- Modeling the way

Case Illustration: Motorola, Inc.   Motorola, Inc., the 1988 Malcolm Baldrige National Quality Award Winner, provides an example of the manager's role in quality through their company's approach to quality as a profitable business strategy. Motorola's managers carry with them the corporate objective of total customer satisfaction—literally. It is on printed cards that they carry in their pockets. Corporate officials and business managers wear pagers to make themselves available to customers, and they regularly visit customers' businesses to find out what they like and don't like about Motorola products and services. This information, along with data gathered through an extensive network of customer surveys, complaint hot lines, field audits, and other customer feedback measures, guides planning for quality improvement and product development.

In response to the rapid rise of Japanese electronics competitors in world markets, Motorola's management began an almost evangelical crusade for quality improvement, addressing it as a company issue and, through speeches and full-page advertisements in major publications, as a national issue. The Motorola management demonstrates its quality leadership in a variety of ways, including top-level meetings to review quality programs with results passed on through the organization. However, employees at all levels of the company are also involved. Employees contribute directly through Motorola's Participative Management Program (PMP). Composed of employees who work in the same area or who are assigned to achieve a specific goal, PMP teams meet often to assess progress toward meeting quality goals, to identify new initiatives, and to work on problems. To reward high-quality work, savings that stem from team recommendations are shared. PMP bonuses over the past four years have averaged about three percent of Motorola's payroll.

Managers also ensure that employees have the skills necessary to achieve company objectives. This is accomplished through the training center that Motorola set up, a center through which they spent more than $170 million on worker education between 1983 and 1987. About 40 percent of the training the company provided last year was devoted to quality matters, ranging from general principles of quality improvement to designing for manufacturability.

Moreover, Motorola's leaders know what levels of quality their products must achieve to top their competitors. Each of the firm's six major groups and sectors have benchmarking programs that analyze all aspects of a competitor's products to assess their manufacturability, reliability, manufacturing cost, and performance. Motorola has measured the products of about 125 companies against its own standards, verifying that many Motorola products rank best in their class.

Lessons Learned   The lessons learned for middle managers from the Motorola illustration include the following:

- Recognizing the critical role of customer access and constantly gathering customer knowledge for use in planning, improvement, and development of new products and services
- Engaging employees in decision making and improvement to support a culture of involvement
- Providing incentives that reward and recognize participation and improvement
- Actively participating in the process when needed to advance the work rather than coming in at the end to judge "go or no go" on an initiative, a strategy that will eliminate bureaucracy and increase meaningful participation

- Providing the resources for employee training and development that is strategically focused to help people improve in areas that matter to the company's success
- Establishing expectations to achieve best-in-class performance through external benchmarking and rigorously measuring and communicating performance to employees to provide focus and hold people accountable for actions at the front line

Quality Professionals

There has been a change in the role of many quality professionals. This change requires that there be a staff function to guide the development of governance and management abilities to lead in the quality process. It also includes consulting throughout the organization to nurture the attitude of inquiry, the passion to serve customers, and the advancement of the employees' skills to perform well as individuals and in teams. Such a role requires a clear and tough-minded insistence on recognizing and responding to customer requirements and preferences and on providing the organization with critical performance measures and best-in-class targets that can drive strategy, rate of change, and operating results. Quality professionals focus attention of the organization on improvement, ensuring that the infrastructure exists so that all employees can contribute fully. Coaching leaders is also a key role function. Scanning the organization, the quality professional can identify areas of performance that need improvement as well as identify better practices to promote learning. Figure 1-1 shows a mission statement of a quality function reflecting the changing role described.

Case Illustration: GTE   The role of the quality professional as a coach, facilitator, and expert resource is illustrated through the approach to quality used by GTE Directories. The operations of GTE Directories Corporation are driven by a comprehensive, continuous focus on customer satisfaction that combines market research with clear-cut quality improvement processes and techniques. GTE Directories Corporation is in the advertising business and has been a leading Yellow Pages publisher for more than 50 years. In the 1980s, the company began to face competition from other publishers and media that were moving to enter the advertising niche previously reserved for Yellow Pages publishers. With a slowing economy, businesses were increasingly replacing historic faith in advertising with

FIGURE 1-1. Sample Quality Professionals'
Mission Statement

The value quality brings to the organization is the system perspective
and expertise to do the following:

- Provide governance and operations leaders with evidence-based decision support
- Build the structure, processes, and capabilities to reduce error and waste and to make improvement happen
- Apply measurement technology to demonstrate results of performance and gauge change in areas of strategic and operational importance to the organization's purpose
- Design pilots to test innovations in care and service
- Develop and deliver dissemination and education strategies linked to critical areas of performance

Reprinted, with permission, from Allina Health System, Minnetonka, Minn., 1998.

a demand for proof that advertising worked. It was a wake-up call
for GTE.

The response: GTE responded by transforming itself from an organization that relied on experience, enthusiasm, and the gut instincts of an aggressive sales force to a company focused on anticipating and satisfying customer needs, based on concrete, systematic customer input and rigorous quality processes. The company introduced formal quality improvement techniques into its management mainstream in 1986. Quality professionals coached the company's senior management so that they could assume a highly visible leadership role in quality. The senior managers attended quality improvement courses taught by quality professionals; the managers then taught a similar course to more than 400 managers and employees. Quality professionals prepared improvement teams to address business issues using the basic philosophies, tools, and techniques of continuous quality improvement. Action plans developed by the first teams evolved into the company's initial strategic quality plan. Since 1991, GTE has used the Baldrige Award Criteria to drive its internal self-assessment and improvement process. The company uses a comprehensive, disciplined approach to anticipate, meet, and exceed customer needs. The Customer Satisfaction Measurement Program provides quantitative data on customer perceptions of the company's performance. The company vision is "100% customer satisfaction through quality." Quality professionals guide and senior managers lead the company toward this vision.

GTE puts a high value on constantly measuring, reviewing, and refining its processes for operational data. To ensure that data are relevant, customer priorities are used to set company goals and determine what measures will be used. Quality staff members are expert at measurement. To ensure that measurement data are current and relevant, functional and cross-functional process management teams were formed throughout the company to continually review the data. In fact, the team approach is pervasive in the company. Employees use improvement teams to identify problems and change work processes. It is common for an individual to have served on 10 or more teams, and virtually every employee serves on at least 1 team a year. The company also has permanent process management teams that continually monitor and improve core business and support processes. Managers are, in fact, skilled quality professionals.

GTE uses competitive comparisons and benchmarks to compare itself with best-in-class companies against six broad performance categories: customer, products, operations, employees, supplier performance, and core business processes. Service standards are set and measured based on identified customer requirements.

The results: The hardwiring of quality as a core business strategy produced results. The company rates best-in-class for error rates, and the number of advertisers managed by individual sales representatives has increased each year. At the same time, the time spent by each representative with advertisers has increased, one of the documented customer requirements.

The company directories are preferred in 217 of its 274 primary markets, and revenue growth has been sustained. GTE, meanwhile, continues to pursue the vision of 100% customer satisfaction.

Lessons Learned   For quality professionals, the lesson from GTE Directories Corporation is the power of integrating the skills of quality improvement into the mainstream of the organization. Coaching senior management to visibly lead quality would show all employees that skills in improvement were a required performance competency.

Quality was clearly not optional. Quality professionals ensure that the voice of the customer is present throughout the organization through rigorous and systematic measurement. Measures can then be used by content experts to drive the changes for necessary improvement. Managers who model and teach quality principles and skills become quality improvement practitioners and resources for quality in the company. Quality professionals advise, consult, and support the leader's role in creating an environment of quality practice.

INCORPORATE QUALITY PRINCIPLES INTO PERSONAL AND PROFESSIONAL LIFE

For leaders, quality extends beyond application to the organization's business—beyond responsibilities and roles. Quality is a concept that can and should be applied to their personal behavior and beliefs. In the book Quality is Personal, Harry Roberts and Bernard Sergesketter offer challenges to consider in incorporating quality principles into all aspects of a leader's personal and professional life. These principles are guided by four basic ideas.[24] Leaders should do the following:

1. Orient all efforts toward delighting customers and removing waste in internal processes
2. Stress team effort at all levels, inside and outside the organization, including cooperative efforts with suppliers and customers
3. Use data and scientific reasoning to guide and evaluate improvement methods and to hold the gains from past improvements
4. Apply these principles in personal life to improve relationships, increase efficiency, and eliminate waste in all forms

Simple notions are stressed, such as eliminating waste from personal schedules and activities, staying close to the customer, thinking systemically, seeing events in context over time, keeping focused and setting priorities based on the focus, and reflecting and learning from experience. The authors provide guidance on how leaders can understand quality by improving their own methods of prioritizing and organizing and by improving the processes by which they live and work.

Roberts and Sergesketter provide a framework for understanding quality through personal application: The Personal Quality Checklist (figure 1-2).[25] This checklist involves keeping track of shortcomings, or defects, in your key personal work processes. A variation on the approach is to keep track of cycle times. Cycle time is the length of time it takes to go through a process once; for example, the cycle time of a diagnostic test is the elapsed time from when a physician orders a test to when the results are received for decision making. The aim is to reduce both defects and cycle times for important personal processes. The number of defects in your processes cannot be reduced if they are not counted, and cycle time cannot be reduced if it is not measured. This begins the basics of quality improvement: a process, a goal, and measurement over time.

FIGURE 1-2. Personal Quality Checklist

Defect Category	Mon	Tue	Wed	Thu	Fri	Sat	Sun	Total
Late for meeting or appointment								
Search for something misplaced or lost								
Delayed return of phone call or reply to letter								
Putting a small task in a "hold pile"								
Failure to discard incoming junk promptly								
Missing a chance to clean up junk in office								
Unnecessary inspection								
Total								

Comments:

Reprinted with the permission of The Free Press, a Division of Simon & Schuster from *Quality Is Personal: A Foundation for Total Quality Management* by Harry V. Roberts and Bernard F. Sergesketter. Copyright © 1993 by Harry V. Roberts and Bernard F. Sergesketter.

Roberts and Sergesketter suggest getting started by identifying the processes you personally use to do your work. Almost everyone uses meetings, telephone calls, and correspondence in one way or another. Also, it is important for everyone to make a good appearance and to stay healthy. With these factors in mind, in the spring of 1990, Sergesketter developed an initial checklist as a simple way to improve personal quality:[26]

- Be on time for meetings
- Answer phone in two rings or less
- Return phone calls same or next day
- Respond to letters in five business days
- Keep a clean desk
- Have only same day paper on credenza
- Never need a haircut
- Always have shoes shined
- Always have clothes pressed

- Keep weight below 190 pounds
- Exercise at least three times per week

Sergesketter then shared this list with his work associates at AT&T and asked them to help him avoid these defects. He also encouraged associates to start their own lists based on the work they did and what was most important to them. Many did that, and they started to learn more about quality together. The utility of this personal approach becomes clear when the information is compiled[27]:

- *Be on time for meetings:* There is no distinction between major defects and minor defects. If you are one second late, that is a defect. An additional defect can be counted for each minute or five minutes late. Soon, everyone was on time for every meeting. He reported that most people arrived a few minutes early, so many meetings began before the scheduled time. Everyone was there for one 8:00 AM meeting by 7:50 AM, and so the meeting started. It took nine minutes and was over before it was scheduled to begin! The experience has been that meetings take one-third less time when they start promptly. The productivity improvement is enormous, and it costs nothing to achieve.
- *Answer phone in two rings or less:* The aim is to answer the phone in one ring or less. Research has shown that most people think that the phone should be answered in two rings. It was learned from AT&T manufacturing experience that the designed cycle time for a process must be one-half the targeted maximum to have essentially all actual times within the maximum. This gave a chance to teach a quality guideline in a form that could be easily understood and appreciated.
- *Return phone calls the same or next business day:* This is common courtesy and most people think they do an excellent job here, until they start to record the defects. (An appropriate standard is to record an additional defect for each additional day that a call is not returned.)
- *Respond to letters in five business days:* This factor could not be scored until date stamping was set up for all arriving correspondence. Then it took a couple of months to realize that it was necessary to design a process with a mean response of 2.5 days to achieve a nearly 100 percent response in five days.
- *Keep a clean desk and have only same day paper on credenza:* Until "just-in-time" operation is achieved with paper flow,

time is being wasted by going through the same paper without taking any action. All the time spent in prioritizing is wasted. This is another productivity bonus that cost nothing to achieve!

- *Never need a haircut:* You look in the mirror and see that you need a haircut and it can be a week before you can arrange it in your schedule. Charge a defect for each day that you look in the mirror and are dissatisfied with the image on the basis of haircut. One solution is to schedule a haircut on a regular basis. If a haircut is obtained before needed one, then one will never be needed. (This is an insight from Disney World, where there is never a dirty window because they literally wash the windows before the windows get dirty. Prevention achieved through planning is the quality principle.)
- *Always have shoes shined and clothes pressed:* These are similar to the haircut category.
- *Keep weight below 190 pounds:* (This is five pounds above what the charts say is the ideal weight for Sergesketter, who is 6' 5" tall.) One key to success is to manage caloric intake, which illustrates the quality principle that desired results are achieved by working on the processes that produce the results.
- *Exercise at least three times per week:* To achieve fitness in limited time, Sergesketter recommends the Royal Canadian Air Force (RCAF) exercises, which take little time, require no special equipment, and are graduated by age. However, there are other alternatives.

CONCLUSION

Whether the attention is being focused on these personal manifestations of an individual's approach to quality or on the leader's impact on the quality processes of an entire organization, it is the recognition of the leader's crucial role in promoting quality as an essential business strategy that will lead to an organization's success. Figure 1-3 summarizes the findings of the author about the attributes of quality leaders. Having spent this chapter exploring the personal commitment and roles of leadership, the following chapters discuss critical elements, models, and tactics for embedding quality as a strategy within the organization.

FIGURE 1-3. Attributes of Quality Leaders

- Demonstrate personal passion about mission and values
- Embody and inspire quality
- Possess humility/disclosure/inquiry
- Are customer-focused: all activities are linked to customer and mission
- Ensure voice of the customer through personalized contact and stories
- Make clear that quality is not optional
- Set rigorous standards
- Require ongoing measurement and feedback against standards
- Act when necessary to preserve and hold high:
  - Standards
  - Values
- Create truth-telling culture
  - Mistakes/risks
  - Zero tolerance for cover-ups
- Hold central values, managed locally, respectful of norms
- Are data-driven
- Create safe place for conflict and respect of differing perspectives
- Empower others to act
- Connect front office—front line

Reprinted, with permission, from Allina Health System, Minnetonka, Minn., 1998.

References

1. Wennberg, J. E., and A. Gittelsohn, "Small Area Variations in Health Care Delivery," *Science* 182 (Dec. 14, 1973): 1102–8.

2. Leape, L., et al., "Preventing Medical Injury," *Quarterly Review Bulletin* (May 1993): 144–9.

3. Wind, J. Y., and J. Main, *Driving Change: How the Best Companies Are Preparing for the 21st Century* (New York: The Free Press, 1998).

4. Presidential Advisory Commission on Consumer Protection and Quality in the Health Care Industry.

5. Lear, R., "Asking the Right Questions," *Chief Executive* 98 (Oct., 1994): 1–10.

6. Senge, P., "The Leader's New Work: Building Learning Organizations," *Sloan Management Review* 32, no. 1 (Fall, 1990): 7.

7. Senge, p. 7.

8. Senge, p. 7.

9. Senge, p. 9.

10. Treacy, M., *The Discipline of Market Leaders* (New York: Addison–Wesley, 1996).

11. Senge, p. 8.

12. Paulson, P., and Paulson and Associates, Inc. "Bridging Researcher and Practice," Dissemination Conference, Minneapolis, Sept., 1997.

13. DeLavigne, K. T., and J. D. Robertson, *Deming's Profound Changes: When Will the Sleeping Giant Awaken* (New Jersey: PTR Prentice Hall, 1994).

14. Batalden, P. B., and P. K. Stoltz, "A Framework for the Continual Improvement of Health Care: Building and Applying Professional and Improvement Knowledge to Test Changes in Daily Work," *Journal of Performance Improvement in Health Care Organizations* 19, no. 10 (Oct., 1993): 424–52.

15. Batalden, 424–52.

16. "Eyes on the Prize," *Forbes* 145, no. 3 (Feb. 5, 1990): 14(1).

17. Broadhead, J. L., "The Post-Deming Diet: Dismantling a Quality Bureaucracy," *Training: The Magazine of Human Resources Development* 28, no. 2 (Feb., 1991): 41(3).

18. Weisendanger, B., "Deming's Luster Dims at Florida Power and Light," *Journal of Business Strategy* 14, no. 5 (Sept.–Oct., 1993): 60(2).

19. "The Cracks in Quality," *The Economist* 323, no. 7755 (Apr. 18, 1992): 67(2).

20. "Eyes on the Prize," p. 14.

21. Broadhead, p. 41.

22. Broadhead, p. 41.

23. Medtronic Inc. Mission Statement, Minneapolis, Minn.

24. Roberts, H. V., ad B. F. Sergesketter, *Quality is Personal: A Foundation for Total Quality Management* (New York: The Free Press, 1993).

25. Roberts and Sergesketter, pp. 7–12.

26. Roberts and Sergesketter, p. 10.

27. Roberts and Sergesketter, p. 25.

Suggested Readings

Allina Blueprint for Quality (Minnetonka, Minn.: Allina Health System, 1995).

Bennis, W., and P. W. Biederman, *Organizing Genius* (Reading, Mass.: Addison-Wesley, 1997).

Bennis, W., et al., *Leadership in a New Era* (San Francisco: New Leaders Press, 1994).

Berwick, D., "Quality Comes Home," *Quality Connection* 4, no. 1 (Winter, 1995): 1–4.

Berwick, D., A. Blanton Godfrey, and J. Roessner, *Curing Health Care: New Strategies for Quality Improvement* (San Francisco: Jossey-Bass, 1990).

Block, P., *Stewardship* (San Francisco: Berrett-Koehler, 1993).

Collins, J., and J. L. Porras, "Building Your Company's Vision," *Harvard Business Review* 74, no. 3 (Sept.–Oct., 1996): 65–77.

Cooper, R. K., and A. Sawaf, *Executive EQ: Emotional Intelligence in Leadership and Organizations* (New York: Grosset/Putnam, 1996).

Crosby, P. B., *Quality Is Free: The Art of Making Quality Certain* (New York: McGraw Hill, 1979).

Dartmouth Atlas of Health Care, Dartmouth Medical School, the Center for Evaluative Clinical Sciences (Chicago: American Hospital Publishing, 1996).

Fritz, R., *Creating* (New York: Ballantine Books, 1991).

Fukuyama, F., *Trust—The Social Virtues and Creation of Prosperity* (New York: The Free Press, 1995).

Hayward, S., *Churchill on Leadership: Executive Success in the Face of Adversity* (Rocklin, Calif.: Forum: An Imprint of Prima Publishing, 1997).

Heskett, J., W. E. Sasser, and C. Hart, *Service Breakthroughs: Changing the Rules of the Game* (Free Press, Management of Service Operations, 1990).

Heskett, J., W. E. Sasser, and L. A. Schlesinger, *The Service Profit Chain* (New York: The Free Press, 1997).

Hesselbein, F., M. Goldsmith, and R. Beckhard, *Leader of the Future* (San Francisco: Jossey-Bass, 1996).

Johns, T. O., and W. E. Sasser, Jr., "Why Satisfied Customers Defect," *Harvard Business Review* 73, no. 6 (Nov.–Dec., 1995): 88.

Orlikoff, J., and M. K. Totten, *The Board's Role in Quality Care: A Practical Guide for Hospital Trustees* (Chicago: American Hospital Publishing, 1991).

Payne, S., *The Art of Asking Questions* (Princeton, NJ: Princeton University Press, 1980).

Reichheld, F. F., and W. E. Sasser, Jr., "Zero Defections: Quality Comes to Services," *Harvard Business Review* 68, no. 7 (Sept.–Oct., 1990): 105.

Russo, J. E., and P. J. H. Schoemaker, *Decision Traps* (Simon & Schuster, 1990).

Shortell, S., "High-Performing Healthcare Organizations: Guidelines for the Pursuit of Excellence," *Hospital & Health Services Administration* (July–Aug., 1985): 7–33.

Vinten, G., "The Art of Asking Questions," *Management Decision* 32, no. 9 (Dec. 15, 1994): 46(4).

Wennberg, J. E., "Variations in Medical Practice and Hospital Costs," *Connecticut Medicine* 49, no. 7 (1985): 444–535.

Wennberg, J. E., and A. Gittelsohn, "Small Area Variations in Health Care Delivery," *Science* 182 (Dec., 14, 1973): 1102–8.

Wennberg, J. E., B. A. Barnes, and M. Zubkoff, "Professional Uncertainty and the Problem of Supplier-Induced Demand," *Social Science and Medicine* 16, no. 7 (1982): 811–24.

Wheatley, M. J., *Leadership and the New Science* (San Francisco: Berrett-Koehler, 1992).

2

Partnering with the Customer

W hat is the right care? How is care most effectively delivered? What is important to customers about their health care? What do health professionals need to know about continually improving care? What constitutes quality? These questions have launched us into a new frontier in understanding the quality of health care. In health care, significant time and resources have been dedicated to quality improvement. Dr. Jonathan Lord, chief operating officer of the American Hospital Association, concludes that the health care industry has spend a lot of resources to make sure that the trains run on time. He poses that the real question to pursue for quality improvement is, are we putting people on the right train for them?[1]

This chapter suggests that the milestone for quality is the participation of the patient, health plan member, and family in the health care system to determine care and service quality and that the challenge for those in health care is to cope with the complex cultural changes this inclusion implies.

THE QUALITY MILESTONE: PATIENT AS PARTNER

"The patient is not an actuarial table. She's your mother."[2] This quote by J. D. Beckham epitomizes the perspective necessary to affect patient participation within the organization. To deliver quality services and care and to improve health, the patient must become *part of the system, not merely have input into the system.* The customer becomes a partner in the planning, delivery, and evaluation for quality. This calls for cultural changes in our health care systems. It implies that the provider and care team create the health care experience in partnership with an informed patient. The creation of an enduring health care experience aimed at improving the health status of the patient through partnership is a milestone of quality. However, this notion requires complex cultural changes in attitudes, processes, and the overall caregiving system.

In response to an industry-wide focus on quality, traditional care boundaries and the structure of provider-patient relationships have been challenged. Historically, care has been provided by experts and in clinics, hospitals, and medical centers. Care was not directed toward providing informed choices, increasing participation, and encouraging independence of the patient, nor systematically monitoring quality indicators over time to drive improvement related to the health care consumer's needs and preferences.

In the ground-breaking book *Through the Patient's Eyes*, Gerteis exploded the myth of "doctor- or clinician-knows-best." Eclipsing the often self-serving use of satisfaction surveys to gauge the quality of our work, Gerteis studied and learned from patients themselves what mattered. Repeatedly, she found that information, choice, participation, coordination of transitions, and knowing that preferences would be respected and honored were the critical measures of satisfaction for patients.[3]

These critical measures underscore the idea that patients are asking to become part of the health system, not passive recipients of its services. Ultimately, it is the customer who determines quality. The dimensions of care that concern patients and that require our attention are shown in table 2-1. This knowledge ushers us toward a new era for understanding quality in health care.

Why should an organization consider making the journey of transforming health care to fully involve the patient? First, it is the right and ethical thing to do. It also makes good business sense. Multiple studies and sources tell us that it is the experience of care that the patient values. It is the experience of care that creates loyalty. It is the experience of care over time that provides the opportunities to improve health status. And it is the experience of care that builds market share.

TABLE 2-1   Dimensions of Care That Matter to Patients

For Inpatients	*For Clinic Patients*
Respect for patient preferences	Respect for patient preferences
Coordination of care	Access
Information and education	Information and education
Physical comfort	
Emotional support	Emotional support
Involvement of family and friends	
Continuity and transition	Continuity and coordination

Source: Copyright © The Picker Institute, Cambridge, Mass.

The following summarizes the findings of one integrated health care system that analyzed the results from focus groups, satisfaction surveys, and consumer interviews and studies. It describes the care experience desired by patients and health plan members in their own words:[4]

- "I get what I need, when I need it, easily."
- "I am a knowledgeable partner in my health care."
- "I am pleasantly surprised by my experience."
- "I believe the system and its staff are competent."
- "I am respected as an individual and treated with dignity."
- "I feel safe and secure."

Quality as defined by the customer is often a startling assertion to clinicians who have dedicated their professional careers to providing clinical quality in their practices. To assert that the experience of care and service is the differentiator in determining quality in the eyes of the consumer is not to supplant clinical quality. Quite the contrary: clinical quality is an expected foundation of the care experience.

NEW ROLES AND SKILLS FOR CLINICIANS

As the clinician-patient partnership or counselor–health plan member partnership is explored, clinicians and counselors bear the responsibility of being knowledgeable, current, technically proficient, and skilled in integrating aspects of wellness and care. Patients and members bear the responsibility of entering the partnership as full participants in learning about their health, understanding their risks, advocating for their preferences, exploring options, and reducing their health risks.

There is a greeting in South Africa, described by Lawrence Vander Post, that translates as "I see you."[5] The greeting implies that to be a person means to be acknowledged as an individual and to be in relationships with others. Isn't this what patients are saying to us? "See me," not my diagnosis, my risk, my expected cost per hospital day, diagnosis-related group (DRG) or cost (per member per month [PMPM])—but who I am. What I think, fear, need, and prefer.

Clinicians must move from the expert role in which they are the ones conveying information to others to a role that expands their ability to listen and learn from others. This new role requires partnership skills, aligned incentives, and an environment that supports it. For example, clinics that work on a production model requiring a maximum of 15 minutes per patient visit present a challenge. In this setting, a physician might order an ultrasound for an anxious pregnant mother to reassure her that her baby was fine and explain the rationale for the cost of the technology as follows: The use of ultrasonography is reimbursable; the extra time it would take to understand the young woman's apprehension is not. An opportunity for a partnership between the physician and patient is therefore missed.

THE TOTAL QUALITY EVOLUTION

The evolution from the adaptive learning of our past—from the days of using only retrospective reviews, peer review, satisfaction surveying, outcome studies, and benchmarking—to creating a future of generative learning in which we build on shared understanding, knowledge, and vision can occur only when the customer's voice is an active part of the health care system.

Consider figure 2-1, which follows the evolution of quality from a status quo expert model to a state in which the customer is a partner and part of the system; value is created and managed when contact is made with the customer. From the status quo of expert-knows-best and providing services to a passive recipient (the patient or member), many organizations moved to either a customer service or quality control program. Ultimately, most moved on to an emphasis on quality improvement. In the future, they must progress to total quality.

FIGURE 2-1.   Evolution of Quality in Health Care

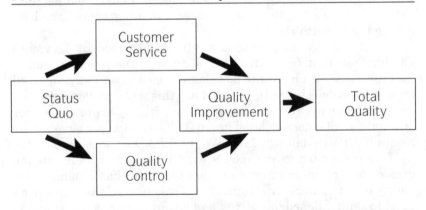

- *Status quo:* Provider knows best. The evolution to total quality developed gradually. The status quo approach was designed for product production in which the product was sent from the organization to the customer. It was a one-way transaction. In our work, the status quo is evident when the clinician provides care or service—our product—to a patient who is a passive recipient, as depicted in figure 2-2. The health plan designs a product, and it is sent to the market place.
- *Customer service model:* This is feedback after the fact. The customer service model is built on the acknowledgment that complaints will occur. It demonstrates a consciousness that there are problems in the product and that defects do occur. The organization builds in ways to deal with problems. In health care, the customer service model acknowledges that problems in care and service—unnecessary variance, failures in process or products—exist in our organizations. Many of us have institutionalized our response to problems in the form of member or patient representatives and other roles and departments. The product is out, and we receive feedback in the form of anecdotal accounts of problems so that we can correct them, as is depicted in figure 2-3.

FIGURE 2-2. Status Quo Model

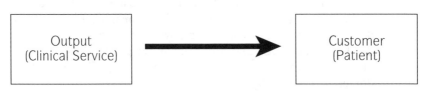

Reprinted, with permission, from Allina Health System, Minnetonka, Minn., 1998.

FIGURE 2-3. Customer Service Model

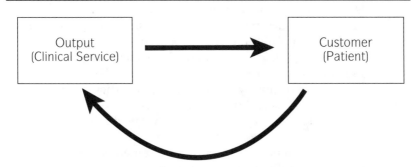

Reprinted, with permission, from Allina Health System, Minnetonka, Minn., 1998.

FIGURE 2-4.   Quality Control Model

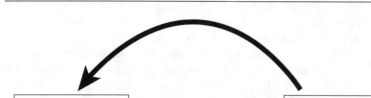

Reprinted, with permission, from Allina Health System, Minnetonka, Minn., 1998.

- *Quality control model:* Feedback is used to set standards. Quality control evolved as a reaction to accumulated customer service complaints. It is a model that assumes people are the problem. It sets standards, measures performance, and catches people and punishes them for not meeting standard performance levels. Often what occurs is that standards are narrowed and higher levels of performance are expected within the systems and structures. This model is depicted in figure 2-4.
- *Continuous quality improvement model:* Improvement is based on ongoing feedback. In the next level of quality evolution, continuous quality improvement (depicted in figure 2-5), the focus is on processes. This level is open to understanding customer requirements as input to the system and is more accommodating of feedback on performance. However, it is often internally focused and not systemic.
- *Total quality:* Customers actively participate in the planning, delivery, and evaluation of care. At the highest level, creating total quality within an organization involves systemic inquiry and partnership. A vision is used to attract and inspire commitment and loyalty. The distinguishing feature in total quality is that it is focused on bringing the customer and the market in, rather than merely getting a product out. In addition, enduring partnerships are valued and nurtured. Value-added products and services are created in

this model, with customer participation and preferences in mind. Caring and service excellence are hallmarks of the organization.

At this level of quality, depicted in figure 2-6, knowledge about patients is acquired through a variety of sources and is applied in

FIGURE 2-5. Continuous Quality Improvement Model

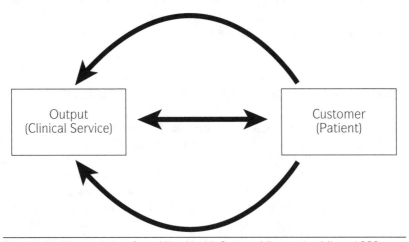

Reprinted, with permission, from Allina Health System, Minnetonka, Minn., 1998.

FIGURE 2-6. Total Quality

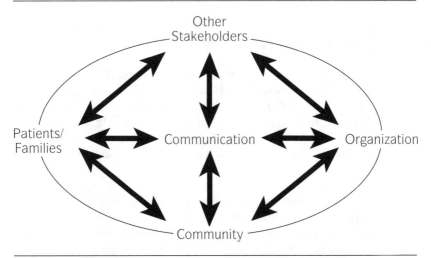

Reprinted, with permission, from Allina Health System, Minnetonka, Minn., 1998.

all aspects of business. Sources include focus groups, consumer-affairs panels, consumer and community boards and committees, and product design structures in which customers are actively involved. A respectful and therapeutic environment is evident, in which patients have access to information and resources and are informed partners with clinicians and the care team in planning for their health. An organization of this type embodies value-based practices and decision making. Shared values exist among patients, and community and organizations are developed to guide practice, support decision making, and help identify areas of potential conflict for which resolution processes are developed. This value-based decision-making practice forms the ethics of the organization.[6]

FRAMEWORK FOR MOVING TO TOTAL QUALITY

For partnership to become a cornerstone for quality, it requires more than clinicians' good intentions and patients' desire to assume greater responsibility for their health and health care decisions. An organizational context or framework needs to be developed in which partnering with patients and families is expected, measured, and rewarded. Bringing the patient into the care system as a full participant must become a normal part of how the organization or system does its work rather than an optional exercise. The processes of providing care and designing support systems must be based on a knowledge of the customer's—the patient's—requirements and preferences.

Planning for the Quality Journey

Donald Berwick authored an important article on this subject, "The Total Customer Relationship in Health Care: Broadening the Bandwidth."[7] He notes that there may be something to learn outside of the health care industry about a "total customer relationship" that can elevate our industry beyond "report cards" and other attempts to determine quality. These relationships include the following elements:

- *Customers as assistants in decreasing waste:* Decreasing waste is demanding work. It means providing only the care and services that the customer needs and eliminating other elements. In health care, many time wasters can be found: movement of supplies; inventory; unused space, equipment, and most paperwork; time that people spend being idle or uncertain about what action to take; and too much administration. In conjunction with the care system, the customer will determine what is needed. This requires listening carefully to what the customer does and does not want and focusing action accordingly.

- *Mass customization and stratification of need:* In best-of-class service companies, customers experience the work as if it were individualized for them. The companies, such as Ritz-Carlton hotels, may not know each customer as a unique individual, but they have a deep understanding of groups of customers in their market. "One-size-fits-all" approaches have been replaced by stratification or identification of specific needs of a group or population and customization of a general approach to that specific population. Through stratification and by delivering care and service by "mass customization," resources can be freed to provide the individual customization required to meet differing individual needs. Populations to consider include seniors, pregnant women, emergency patients, surgical patients, and diabetics; differences in cultures should also be considered.

- *Shaping demand and supporting self-care:* In addition to focusing on meeting customer needs and expectations, health care has an opportunity to work with the customer to shape expectations for care and services. Engaging in a process to work with health plan members and patients about possibilities, alternatives, and expected experiences help shape the patients' behavior when seeking care and services. For example, group education versus repeated individual instruction about a disease state, expected length of hospitalization, self-care strategies for managing chronic disease, and access to care providers other than physicians (such as nurse practitioner or nurse educator) for services are all areas of consideration. Impressive results are being reported in the literature of better outcomes, better service, and lower costs when prepared and informed patients manage their care (for example, diabetics controlling glycosylated hemoglobin and asthmatics controlling their asthma).

- *Immediate recovery:* Immediate recovery is the commitment to keep a promise, with no excuses allowed. In best-of-class companies, recovery that is immediate and thorough recreates and deepens customer loyalty. Health care has just begun to wrestle with the issue of guarantees and promises. For Berwick, immediate recovery offers a vehicle to explore an important question with patients, families, and health plan members as customers: What do we promise, and how do we back up that promise if we fail? Documentation of immediate recovery situations provides a source of information about process failures and customers' needs that informs improvement and innovation. This strategy requires cultural changes in most health care organizations: greater local autonomy to act, support and resources by leaders for use in recovery, and clarity about promises made or implied to the consumer of care.

- *Delight as the objective:* Delighting the customer raises the bar for future performance of the organization. This notion goes far beyond satisfying the expressed needs and expectations for care and service. Delighting the customer challenges health care systems to create and deliver the unexpected experience of care. This requires a deep understanding of the customers: what they hope for, how they live, and what they worry about for their own health and for the health of those close to them. Customers become assets in the organization's learning process when they have the opportunity to talk face-to-face with health care leaders. Satisfaction surveys, report cards, and other instruments currently in use fall short of this exploration for innovation.
- *Customer knowledge and innovation:* Delighting customers by creating surprising experiences responds to latent needs today and shapes expectations for tomorrow's standards of care. This cycle of customer knowledge and redesign of care, service, and product produces the innovations required to resolve the complex issues that health care is currently facing. As Berwick challenges, if leaders and providers persist in believing that our customers have unrealistic expectations about health care experiences—such as relief from pain, access to their doctors, desire to survive cancer, and affordable care—then we deny ourselves the opportunity to invent, innovate, and improve health care.[8]

He included a credo that might guide this development of total customer relationship. It is a reminder to those who the health care system serves of its purpose:

- In a helping profession, the ultimate judge of performance is the person helped.
- Most people, including sick people, are reasonable most of the time.
- Different people have different, legitimate needs.

- Pain and fear produce anxiety in both the victim and the helper.
- Meeting needs without waste is a strategic and moral imperative.[9]

The journey to the milestone of customer involvement starts with a "journey from within" for those who have the ability and responsibility to provide leadership. Each leader, administrative and clinical, needs to address the following questions:

- What leadership model do I follow? What model does my organization follow?
- How do I approach learning about patients' preferences and new care alternatives?
- How do I partner with stakeholders?
- Do I ask questions about others' opinions and consider their answers?
- Do I identify and understand patients' and families' requirements?
- Do I model the changes I hope to see in the health care environment?

These questions help identify where the leader is today and help provide a basis for addressing the steps necessary to achieve a total quality environment.

Assessing the Existing Environment

The leader's role is to create an enabling environment for the organization to move along its quality journey and to create a partnership with the customer. In doing so, some assessment questions need to be asked:

- *What are my current sources of information about customers?* For example: Is there a patient and health plan member satisfaction survey system and complaint system? Do I conduct or attend patient, family, or health plan member focus groups? Do I keep a journal of qualitative information I receive from patients and family members? Do I have community- or constituency-based listening posts in the community at large? Do I have a way for staff members to tell me about their experiences with customers?

- *How do I disseminate and use that information?* For example: Do I routinely talk about customer requirements in staff meetings? Do I have mechanisms to report survey findings? Do I have local (unit-based) hospital or health plan measurements about satisfaction or requirements that are relevant to and can be acted on at the front line? Are educational offerings and curricula built around customer requirements and feedback? How do I convert process failures and complaints into learning or improvement opportunities?
- *What do I ask about, measure, and monitor as a reflection of what I value?* For example: Do my questions focus on budget and workload, or do they address understanding whether care and services are improving? What do I ask about first? How do I phrase my inquiry? Do I recognize the existing performance within my setting as viewed by the customer?
- *How do I spend my time, and how do I stay close to the customer?* For example: Have I arranged my schedule according to what is meaningful and valuable to me? Do I consciously make time to spend time with my customers?
- *How does my calendar of activities reflect a direct contribution to safety and improvement?*
- *What systems do I have in place to ensure that customers' voices are heard in my decision making?* For example: Do I regularly have quantitative and qualitative data available to support decision making? Are the data systematically acquired and analyzed over time to evaluate the results of decision making?
- *What performance and outcome feedback is available to clinicians that is relevant and can be acted on at the front line?* For example: Are there performance profiles that focus on key processes and the outcome measures to be achieved? Are interdisciplinary teams provided with regular feedback on the results of their efforts, including communication with patients and health plan members, informing them about their preferences, and encouraging joint planning of care, benefit decisions, and services?
- *Are measurement and feedback used for learning and improvement?* For example: How do I address staff mistakes, customer complaints, and process failures? Are these events seen as opportunities for learning and improvement? Do I look for improvement over time and across departmental boundaries? Do staff members hear from me only when performance is declining? Do I celebrate learning and improvement? Do I improve my own performance through feedback mechanisms? Is my leadership team improving its methods?

- *What are my vehicles and strategies for compiling or disseminating customer information?* For example: Do I provide and support educational and publishing resources as strategic methods of disseminating and reinforcing partnering strategies? Do I know who the practice and service exemplars are? Do I have mechanisms to tell their stories to staff members? Do consumers participate in meetings or quality improvement teams? Do I have access to and knowledge of how to use technology such as the Internet, public service announcements, and interactive video? Do education strategies reflect customer needs and preferences? Were they created with patients and/or community members? Are translation services or multilingual materials available in visual, auditory, and even kinesthetic presentations? Most important, what investment have I made in developing the skills of employees in listening and consulting and in incorporating customer requirements and preferences in collaborative care decisions and wellness/prevention strategies? What percentage of the salary budget is used for education?

Assessing Customer Needs and Expectations

Research emphasizes the necessity of including customer expectations and enlisting their participation in the health improvement and health care process. There is evidence that doing so improves the physiological outcome of care and the patient's satisfaction. Partnering with the patient is not merely a response to customer demands, it can improve health. J. C. Hornberger, H. Habraken, and D. Bloch concluded that patients want more involvement than ever in decisions affecting their health, and patients who are integral partners in health care decisions are more satisfied with care, adhere more readily to recommendations, and experience better health outcomes.[10]

In his examination of research on patient satisfaction and the factors that influence attitudes in primary care, J. Rees Lewis noted that quality of care is often assessed by provider- or government-derived measures rather than by dimensions patients consider important.[11]

His work challenges organizations formed around "modified paternalism" or "tokenism." For Lewis, listening is a sign of respect and caring. The provider who fails to listen may miss the real concern of the patient and the opportunity to provide care. Patients miss the opportunity to be involved participants in their care and the experience of being cared for.[12]

Research continues to address the issue of what patients want in the area of participation. In her studies of patient partnerships, Raisa Deber makes the distinction that wanting to know is not the same as being in charge.[13] Until that distinction is explored and understood, the roles of the patient and provider will not be clear, and genuine shared decision making will not be possible. She explores the continuum from sensitive paternalism to informed consent and concludes that neither results in shared decision making. To achieve this goal, she suggests that patients and providers need to focus clearly on the following topics and explore each fully in a conversation in language that is understandable and in a setting that allows time to ask questions:

- Available alternatives
- Potential outcomes of each alternative
- Costs, risks, and benefits of each alternative
- Values of each potential outcome

Mutual understanding of and satisfactory agreement on each topic moves the provider-patient relationship to a partnership based on the content of care decisions and plan of care.

EFFECT OF PARTNERSHIP ON COSTS

Many delivery systems are now working with health plans or in integrated health care systems that include financing mechanisms and care management. For them, *demand management* is a term that is gaining significance. The premise of demand management is that health care use and costs will be reduced significantly only when the demand for health care services from the consumer is reduced.[14]

Demand management again raises the issue of patient access to information, counseling, and partnership. It uses decision making and self-management support systems to enable and encourage consumers to make appropriate use of health care resources. It is rational and information based. There is evidence that individuals with access to self-help and self-care have greater confidence in their ability to self-manage and less dependence on health care providers. Individuals who consciously choose healthful lifestyles tend to need less medical care for preventable illnesses.[15] They also are able to exercise informed choice and choose less risky options that tend to be less costly. Dr. John Wennberg and other researchers have convincingly shown that informed patients choose more conservative approaches to care rather than the sites that are identified as benchmarks for low cost and conservative care patterns.[16] The Dartmouth Atlas documents in detail wide variations in health care and draws some provocative conclusions.[17] The authors are cautious not to declare "what care is right" in their analysis of the variation, but they do conclude that the way to determine what is best is to include fully informed consumers in shared decision making with their provider to answer that question.

Access systems need to be designed to encourage customer participation and involvement. They may include consumer service lines, support services, care management systems, and broad-based community programs. Specifically, they may involve the following:

- Nurse-staffed phone lines for information, counseling, and consultations
- Psychosocial support for patients and families who face difficult decisions, including opportunities to rehearse possible scenarios before decisions are necessary, particularly in the area of palliative care and medical futility
- Organized systems (such as a network of health counselors or a case management system) to assist individuals in managing chronic disease; for example, a day planner to track relevant information, medication schedules, physician appointments, physiological parameters (such as glycosylated hemoglobin), and treatment and/or activity regimens to help the patient manage and own his or her care plan, and a journal for keeping track of questions to ask the clinician or suggestions from the clinician
- Health promotion programs and products, including individual risk assessments and immediate feedback on behavior changes to enhance wellness; partnerships with health clubs, schools, and community groups for health education and fitness activities; and dissemination of age-specific U.S. Health Prevention Guidelines, such as environmental risk assessments for infants and toddlers

TOOLS FOR INTERACTING WITH CUSTOMERS

Most health care organizations have focused their energy on sending educational and promotional materials to consumers. There is growing evidence that it might be more helpful and productive for consumers to get materials in ways that are more flexible and interactive.

In addition to the blizzard of consumer-oriented health promotion and health care literature available, other tools such as the Internet, which has the capabilities to search the literature for specific topics and treatment protocols, as well as to access self-care information and advice, are available. Provider-specific and health system–specific home pages in the World Wide Web are available for health-related directories and information. Interactive CD-ROM software provides patients and other consumers decision-support capabilities in considering treatment options and alternatives. Programs for specific condition information and monitoring are available in various languages. Most health care organizations have increased their community education initiatives to include telemedicine and television broadcasts. Also, more and more organizations require or use process and outcome measures to inform the public about general health care, the organization itself, and in some instances, provider- and group-specific performance. Reference libraries and computer access for consumers are becoming common in care sites. Armed with this information, consumers are now asking for comparative information that supports informed choices.

A looming issue rests in the question of how an informed consumer will act in making health care choices. This leads to the idea of creating tools such as report cards that patients can use when selecting physicians, health plans, and hospitals. The theory is that when consumers (patients, employers, or public buyers of health care) have comparative information about the outcomes, costs, and satisfaction associated with different providers, health plans, and delivery systems, they will choose the options that excel. Competition will do the rest to improve quality and contain costs.[18] Although issues of technological capability, safeguarding privacy of patient data, and questions of how data would be released to consumers are the subject of considerable debate, this area continues to warrant attention and development.

We need to monitor and participate in the development of tools that support an informed patient as partner. Measurements used for improving performance can also be used to inform and educate the public. For example, the implementation of Agency for Health Care Policy and Research (AHCPR) guidelines for pressure ulcers, produced in language for both providers and consumers, not only reduced the incidence of pressure ulcers in one health system but also substantially reduced costs, demonstrated accountability to the public for improved outcomes, and provided a vehicle for customer-designed strategies in quality. The Foundation for Accountability (FACCT) is another organization committed to providing consumers with information to support informed choice.

EXEMPLARS IN CUSTOMER PARTNERSHIP

Numerous books that stress the importance of creating a customer focus and bringing the customer voice inside the organization as a strategy for business success and profitability are on the market. The references include *The Discipline of Market Leaders* by Michael Treacy,[19] *The Loyalty Effect* by Fredrich F. Reichheld,[20] and *Winning the Service Game* by Benjamin Schneider and David E. Bowen.[21]

Following are specific illustrations of successful companies noted for quality that have made advancements toward the milestone of bringing the customer voice inside the organization:

ADAC Laboratories

ADAC's whole-organization approach to increasing customer satisfaction and improving quality may be illustrated best by the novel 1993 decision to eliminate the Quality Council, a body composed of executives and managers charged with overseeing the company's quality management process. As a result of benchmarking a Baldrige-winning company, ADAC replaced the council with two weekly meetings that are open to all employees as well as customers and suppliers. During these meetings, numerous employees present data on key measures of customer satisfaction, quality, productivity, and operational and financial performance. Customers engage in discussion and planning.

Corning Telecommunications Products Division

In the rapidly growing global market for optical fiber, the Telecommunications Products Division (TPD) of Corning Inc. aspires to be the best in the industry. TPD already can lay claim to being first in this area because Corning's innovations largely led to the commercialization of optical fiber. Yet, TPD continues to pioneer technology and processes that set it apart from its competitors. Believing that customers are the ultimate judges of what is best, the entire organization is focused on customer satisfaction.

Customer satisfaction is foremost among TPD's key strategic initiatives. Both motivated and guided by feedback received from Baldrige Quality Award examiners in 1989, the company has developed an integrated approach to interacting with existing and prospective customers. TPD's Customer Response System provides the structure for gathering customer inputs, establishing priorities, and initiating action plans to increase levels of customer satisfaction. Input is collected in a variety of ways: surveys, report cards, competitive comparisons, focus groups, and other means of assessing customer satisfaction and perceptions of quality. This information is organized in a customer database that is accessible to all employees. The system provides the means to distill key customer requirements into continuous improvement action plans with measurable critical success indicators.

Custom Research Inc.

Custom Research Inc. (CRI), a national marketing research firm, leverages an intensive focus on customer satisfaction, a team-oriented workforce, and advances in information technology to pursue old-fashioned ends: individualized service and satisfied customers. Since 1988, when CRI adopted its highly focused customer-as-partner approach, client satisfaction has risen from already high levels, and gains in productivity, sales volume, and profits have outpaced industry averages.

CRI's steering committee is responsible for crafting CRI's goals and strategies and views customer loyalty as the firm's most valuable business asset. With all CRI employees as members of customer-focused teams, a flat organizational structure helps make executives immediately accessible to employees, customers, and suppliers. Well-developed systems are in place for understanding customer expectations, soliciting customer feedback, and monitoring each facet of company, team, and individual performance. Together, these systems help set the course for CRI's efforts to meet or exceed customer expectations that can serve as a model for other professional services firms.

Trident Precision Manufacturing Inc.

Founded in 1979, Trident Precision Manufacturing Inc. is a privately held contract manufacturer of precision sheet metal components, electromechanical assemblies, and custom products. The company develops tooling and processes to manufacture components and assemblies designed by its customers in a variety of industries, including office equipment, medical supplies, banking, computers, and defense. The company's 167 employees are based in a single manufacturing facility in Webster, New York.

Regular contact with customers and suppliers is an essential element of Trident's quality strategy. Senior executives meet twice a year with representatives of each customer company for in-depth discussions on Trident's performance as a supplier, and 41 customer-contact personnel interact with these firms daily. Customers, as well as key suppliers, also participate in continuous involvement meetings, initiated by Trident to gain full understanding of a customer's new or modified product design. Direct feedback flags existing and potential problems that can be acted on immediately, and it alerts Trident to changing customer requirements that can be addressed in short- and long-range planning. Responding to future requirements identified through such discussions, for example, Trident recently raised its goal for manufacturing process reliability to a level significantly more stringent than now specified by its most demanding customers.

Abbott Northwestern Hospital

A health care example of this kind of customer involvement is Abbott Northwestern Hospital, a 638-bed acute-care hospital located in Minneapolis, Minnesota, and part of Allina Health System. In 1991, the hospital implemented a personal mastery staff development series. Retreats are held in which principles and skills in mutuality and intentional caring are explored. A key element of the retreat is the interaction with former patients and their families in which they tell their experiences with Abbott Northwestern's care system. Through the patients' eyes and voices, staff members learn which aspects of care and environment were supportive and enabled healing and which aspects did not. Real stories and dialogue with the staff bring the customer inside. The patients and families become faculty, so providers can better understand the experience of care. Charters of Care are developed at these retreats representing the commitments the participants have made to change processes and practices in response to what patients and their families have said they needed and preferred.

The personal mastery experience is available to interdisciplinary teams, and patients are scheduled to meet and talk with the senior leadership about their views of the hospital, its care, and areas for improvement. Direct face-to-face engagement with the customer complements satisfaction surveying, focus groups, and other listening opportunities.

CONCLUSION

As new models of health care emerge and competition in the field increases, the ability to establish meaningful partnerships with customers becomes essential. Failure to establish relationships and partnerships will reduce the ability of organizations to provide customer-driven, value-added care and services and to achieve results.

Society—either as individuals or as demographic groups, populations, and communities—is telling the health care industry that it expects clinical excellence and requires partnerships. Partnerships provide information and support and encourage customer participation in decision making about health and treatment decisions and the creation of services and products. Partnering is the basis of advancing quality of care and fulfilling the obligation of caring.

Partnering with customers also means partnering with the community to understand the complexities of access, community functioning, and support networks. This knowledge is essential to enter the multiple-community, collaborative partnerships needed to improve health and to care for the growing population of aging individuals with one or more chronic health conditions.

Acquiring and using customer knowledge is the basis for service excellence and competitive advantage. Those leaders and health care organizations that are knowledgeable, skilled, and committed to developing effective, sustained partnerships are those that will succeed.

Leadership and the involvement of the customer as part of the system has been outlined. The remainder of this book describes and explores the model, systems, infrastructure, and measurements that leaders must develop in the culture of customer participation and total quality. The patient, health plan member, family, and community are an integral part of the system, not just an input to the system. The social contract for health care is changing to include consumers as fully informed partners in the care process with their providers and the care system. Consumers of health care are redefining the definitions and measures of quality.

No longer satisfied to be a passive recipient of care and services, consumers are demanding to become partners in health care. Doesn't this make sense? It does, yet it changes fundamentally how health care has been defined, planned, organized, delivered, and measured. The health care company that recognizes, designs, and engages the organization in total quality as an intrinsic business strategy will be prepared to change and succeed.

References

1. Lord, J., Comments from presentation, Eye on the Patient: What Care Is Right? Washington, D. C., Oct., 1997, and Seattle, Wash., June, 1998. Sponsored by AHA, AONE, AARP, and Regional Healthcare Associates (Chicago: American Hospital Association, 1997).

2. Beckham, J. D., "The Most Important Day," *Healthcare Forum* 39, no. 3 (May-June, 1996): 84–7, 89.

3. Gerteis M., et al., *Through the Patient's Eyes* (San Francisco: Jossey-Bass Health Series, 1993).

4. Floyd, M., et al., "Service Excellence," *Allina Health Systems, Work of Task Force* (Minnetonka, Minn.: Allina Health System, Nov., 1996).

5. Vander Post, L., Interview, Videotape: *Exemplary Personalities* (Human Dynamics International, 1994).

6. Morath, J., "Thoughts on Ethics and the Art, Science, and Business of Health Care," *Allina Medical Journal* 5, no. 4 (Fall, 1996): 6.

7. Berwick, D., "The Total Customer Relationship in Health Care: Broadening the Bandwidth," *Journal on Quality Improvement* 23, no. 5 (May, 1997): 246.

8. Berwick, p. 246.

9. Berwick, p. 246.

10. Hornberger, J. C., H. Habraken, and D. Bloch, "Minimum Data Needed in Patient Preferences for Accurate, Efficient Medical Decision Making," *Medical Care* 33, no. 3 (1995): 297–310.

11. Lewis, J. R., "Patient Views in Quality Care in General Practice: Literature Review," *Social Sciences Medicine* 39, no. 5 (1994): 655–70.

12. Lewis, pp. 655–70.

13. Deber, R. B., "Physicians in Healthcare Management: The Patient-Physician Partnership. Decision Making, Problem Solving, and the Desire to Participate," *Canadian Medical Association Journal* 151, no. 4 (1994): 423–7.

14. Vickery, D. M., and W. D. Lynch, "Demand Management: Enabling Patients to Use Medical Care Appropriately," *Journal of Occupational and Environmental Medicine* 37, no. 5 (May, 1995): 551.

15. Vickery and Lynch, p. 551.

16. Kasper, J. F., A. G. Mulley, Jr., and J. E. Wennberg, "Developing Shared Decision-Making Programs to Improve the Quality of Health Care," *Quality Review Bulletin* (June, 1992): 183–90.

17. Center for Evaluative Clinical Science, Department of Medical School, *The Department Atlas of Health Care in the United States*, 1998 edition (Chicago: American Hospital Publishing, 1998).

18. Baumgarten, J. D. M. A., "How will consumers use report cards in selecting health plans?" *Managed Care Quarterly* 3, no. 4 (1995): 32–5.

19. Treacy, M., *The Discipline of Market Leaders* (New York: Addison-Wesley, 1996).

20. Reichheld, F. F., *Loyalty Effect: The Hidden Force Behind Growth Profit and Lasting Value* (Boston: Harvard Business School Press, 1996).

21. Schneider, B., and D. E. Bowen, *Winning the Service Game* (New York: McGraw Hill, 1995).

Suggested Readings

Eddy, D. M., "The Individual vs. Society: Is There a Conflict?" *Journal of the American Medical Association* 265, no. 11 (Mar. 20, 1991): 1446, 1449–50.

Eddy, D. M., "The Individual vs. Society: Resolving the Conflict," *Journal of the American Medical Association* 265, no. 18 (May 8, 1991): 2399–401.

Fischhoff, B., and J. Downs, "Accentuate the Relevant," *Psychological Science* 8, no. 3 (May, 1997): 154–8.

Hart, C. W. L., J. L. Heskett, and W. E. Sasser, Jr., "The Profitable Art of Service Recovery," *Harvard Business Review* 68, no. 4 (July-Aug., 1990): 148(9).

Heskett, J. L., et al., "Putting the Service-Profit Chain to Work," *Harvard Business Review* 72, no. 2 (Mar.-Apr., 1994): 164(11).

Heymann, J., "Providing Patients the Information They Need," *Journal of Quality Improvement* 2, no. 8 (1997): 443.

Jones, T. O., and W. E. Sasser, Jr., "Why Satisfied Customers Defect," *Harvard Business Review* 73, no. 6 (Nov.-Dec., 1995): 88(12).

Morath, J., *Patient as Partner: The Cornerstone of Community Health Improvement, AONE Leadership Series, American Organization of Nurse Executives* (Chicago: American Hospital Publishing, 1997).

Nolan, T. W., and L. P. Provost, "Understanding Variation," *Quality Progress* 23, no. 5 (May, 1990): 70–8.

Reichheld, F. F., and W. E. Sasser, Jr., "Zero Defections: Quality Comes to Services," *Harvard Business Review* 68, no. 5 (Sept.-Oct., 1990): 105(7).

Wheeler, D. J., *Understanding Variation* (Knoxville: SPC Press, 1993).

Wheelwright, S. C., and W. E. Sasser, Jr., "The New Product Development Map," *Harvard Business Review* 67, no. 3 (May-June, 1989): 112(10).

3

Reducing Errors and Increasing Safety

The creed of nurses, physicians, and in fact, all health care providers follows Florence Nightingale's dictum—first, do no harm.[1] In health care, accidents and errors mean harm is being done to the patient, the organization is wasting money and resources, and consumers are losing confidence and respect for the organization.

This chapter looks at the tasks involved in reducing accidents and errors and discusses the role of leadership and why errors occur. It also examines lessons learned from other industries and offers a picture of a high-reliability organization.

ACTIONS FOR REDUCING ACCIDENTS AND ERRORS

Reducing the number of accidents and errors is a basic task. It is the job of leaders to declare that error reduction is the foundation of quality improvement.

Create a Safe Place to Examine Errors

The first task is to create a safe place to examine accidents, errors, and untoward events. Reporting them is an obligation so that information can be gathered, studied, and used to predict and prevent future errors. In a quality culture, in which care and services are consistently reliable, there is no room for a search for bad apples and any subsequent punishment. Such behavior drives data underground, shuts down communication, and denies learning and improvement.

Look at Processes and Systems

As health care has become more complex and less based on the individual, more coordination and attention to process is required. By examining what constitutes cooperation and seeking to understand the design and execution of a process, an organization can move closer to being able to (1) appreciate the issue of accidents and errors, (2) create a safe environment to talk about accidents and errors, (3) understand why accidents and errors occur, (4) gain knowledge and expertise in predicting and avoiding accidents and errors, and in so doing, (5) move closer to a responsibility of ensuring a safe place to receive and give care.

This is not easy material. Understanding the processes and systems required is complex, but experts are available to help. To gain appreciation for the depth of this topic, a recommended starting point is Donald Norman's *The Psychology of Everyday Things*.[2] This book leaves one aware of the enormous vulnerability to error and failure that patients and providers confront just by being human, when facing processes and systems that affect them in health care interactions.

Embrace Error Reduction as a Business Imperative

If the reduction of accidents and errors is embraced as a business imperative, then errors need to be examined in enormous detail. The organization—not the individual—must be examined from a process flow perspective, with the individual being viewed as an element in a complex system that led to error. In most organizations, people have learned to work around complexity, procedure failure, and other system issues. When their compensatory abilities break down, error occurs. Observe any patient care area. Ask yourself, is it hard to do the wrong thing? For example: How many pharmaceutical agents are packaged the same? Is there evidence of people adapting their practice around faulty systems? For example, is there masking tape by a switch or control mechanism with a message such as, "NEVER TOUCH THIS"?

Norman provides an everyday example of this with the following story:

A friend kindly let me borrow his car. Just before I was about to leave, I found a note waiting for me: "I should have mentioned that to get the key out of the ignition, the car needs to be in reverse." The car needs to be in reverse! If I hadn't seen the note, I never could have figured that out. There was no visible cue in the car: the knowledge for this trick had to reside in the head. If the driver lacks that knowledge, the key stays in the ignition forever.[3]

This is an example of an individual's adaptation to a faulty system. Furthermore, that adaptation is implicit knowledge held in the individual's head. Is there evidence on the observed unit that certain individuals are required to be on duty for things to work or errors to be avoided? Is there evidence of singularly focused staff members performing isolated duties?

Recognize the Work Involved

An important point for leaders to understand is that creating safety in health care is work. It is not that complex delivery sites are designed and built for safety and the people erode it; instead, it is really that people are constantly working to overcome existing faulty design in systems to safeguard safety.

To reduce accidents and errors, the leaders of the organization need to have answers to the following questions:

- Is this a safe place to receive and give care?
- What are our responsibilities to ensure the safety of patients and employees?
- Does our culture allow employees to tell the truth about errors and near misses?
- Do we have the necessary expertise to systematically examine, predict, and eliminate potential for error?

Consider the Culture of Health Care

The movement toward total quality management with its emphasis on improvement, communication, and learning has the risk of subordinating the focus on a hospital's fundamental obligation to provide safe care and services. If the CEO does not appreciate the importance of the issue of safety, the basics needed to achieve a safe place for care are compromised.

Consider the culture in health care. The notion of error is laden with meaning for providers. Historically, errors have been identified as individual human failures, and consequences have centered around negative sanctions or punishment, including legal action. As a result, errors have not been talked about explicitly, data have not been available, and scientific methods have not been applied consistently and systematically to study and understand the reasons behind error. The introduction of continuous quality improvement came as relief. Health care looked at data systems and ways to make improvements in processes, not ways to fix blame. However, today, the issues of safety and error still tend to be dealt with one at a time and managed through a legal risk management channel, separate from the work of improvement.

Making the basics of safety and accident or error reduction explicit strengthens the foundation of quality. Yet making these reductions is a complex issue—strategically, culturally, and technically.

First, if accidents and errors are not an issue that the board of directors and senior executives ask about, they do not carry strategic importance. Second, the issue of reducing accidents and errors raises questions about the deep emotional content of health care work and the sense of failure, guilt, and shame that develop when errors occur. The culture of health care systemically discourages critical evaluation of processes and the failures associated with error. Yet most individual providers worry every day about making mistakes.

Today in health care, work is done in a culture of guilt, in a punitive legal and regulatory environment, and in a context of public opinion that calls for heads to roll when mistakes occur, not for process improvement. The message of this chapter is not about managing individual performance and cautioning people to be more careful, but about aggressively and systematically addressing flawed procedures and processes that create the potential for error.

THE CASE FOR ERROR REDUCTION AS A BUSINESS IMPERATIVE

A commonly cited study originally published in the *Journal of the American Medical Association* attributed 198,000 deaths per year to error in American hospitals.[4] This statistic requires further explanation. Although the adverse event was the proximal cause of death, many of the patients in the referenced study were extremely ill and would have died even if the event had not occurred. The study estimated, however, that about half the deaths resulted from an adverse event that could have been prevented. That means that approximately 100,000 deaths could have been prevented per year.[5] This is more than double the deaths that occur in highway accidents in the

United States each year. It is estimated that $8.6 billion dollars is the cost of preventable adverse events in hospitals.[6] And that is just the tip of the iceberg.

A recent study by Johnson and Bootman,[7] published in the *Archives of Internal Medicine*, asked panels of practicing pharmacists to estimate health care costs associated with unresolved or unrecognized drug-related problems in ambulatory care settings. The calculated estimate was $76.6 billion, with a considerable range from $30.1 billion to $136.8 billion annually. Their analysis of the issue lead to the conclusion that $45.6 billion in morbidity and mortality costs are due to system failures and are therefore preventable.[8]

Few of the adverse events in hospitals are caused by unusual or rare circumstances, which means that most are predictable.[9] The adverse events are familiar: wound infection, drug overdose, wrong drug, insulin reaction, bleeding from anticoagulants, missed diagnoses, falls, and so on.

Iatrogenic injury from adverse events is not new. It has long been recognized as a cause of mortality and morbidity in hospitalized patients. Dr. Lucian Leape, an investigator on this topic, reported that an estimated 4 percent of hospitalized patients were subject to an adverse event.[10] Further study identified that more than two-thirds of those adverse events are preventable.[11] To calibrate the scope of this issue, if the study rates are applied to the United States as a whole, 1,347,000 people suffered iatrogenic injury each year, 938,000 of which were preventable.

A preventable injury implies that methods are known for averting the injury but that the adverse event occurs from a failure to apply what is known. Dr. Leape takes care to define the spectrum of failure.[12] On one end of the spectrum, injuries occur from negligence. In this situation, standards of care, expected norms of treatment, and procedures for safety are well known, as are the probable consequences if they are not followed. Failure to conform to the known standard is an egregious mistake. On the other end of the spectrum, Dr. Leape describes injuries that result from minor errors such as forgetting a laboratory report or misreading a medication dosage.[13] Most injuries from adverse events and most preventable errors are not the result of negligence.[14,15] The Harvard Medical Practice Study further found that the site of care was not significant in an error's preventability. That is, there was no significant difference in overall preventability between adverse events occurring in a hospital, clinic, emergency department, or free-standing ambulatory care unit.[16] Figure 3-1 displays four classifications of adverse events resulting from error.

FIGURE 3-1. Types of Error

Diagnostic
- Error in diagnosis or delay in diagnosis
- Failure to use indicated tests
- Use of outmoded tests or therapy
- Failure to act on the results of monitoring or testing

Treatment
- Technical error in the performance of an operation, procedure, or test
- Error in administering the treatment (including preparation for treatment or operation)
- Error in the dosage of a drug or in the method of using a drug
- Avoidable delay in treatment or in responding to an abnormal test
- Inappropriate (not indicated) care (considering the patient's disease, its severity, and comorbidity, the anticipated benefit from treatment did not significantly exceed the known risk, or a superior alternative treatment was available)

Preventive
- Failure to provide indicated prophylactic treatment
- Inadequate monitoring or follow-up of treatment

Other
- Failure in communication
- Equipment failure
- Other systems failure

Reprinted, with permission, from: L. L. Leape, A. G. Lawthers, T. A. Brennans, and W. G. Johnson, "Preventing Medical Injury," *Quality Review Bulletin* 19 (May, 1993): 144–9(5).

WHY PREVENTABLE ADVERSE EVENTS OCCUR

There are many reasons why adverse events occur, and complexity of the system is clearly one of them. Although doctors, nurses, pharmacists, and other health care workers are careful people, mistakes occur. Even a small error rate can have serious consequences. The one single factor that can be used to predict errors is the number of interventions, which increase the opportunity for error.

Take, for example, medication administration. The average patient receives 10 different medications during a hospitalization.[17] A large teaching hospital (600 beds) may administer close to 4 million doses per year, with each dose creating an opportunity for error. As

Dr. Leape calculated, even if a system is 99.9 percent error free, more than 4,000 errors will occur annually in that hospital. Furthermore, if only 1 percent results in an adverse event, 40 adverse events will be caused from medications alone and will affect people receiving and providing care.

Now, reflect on all the tests, procedures, and treatments that occur not only within the hospital but across the care continuum. It does not take long to identify the potential, the vulnerabilities, and even the trajectories for error to occur in the health care experience.

DEFINITION OF ERROR

David Woods, from the Institute for Ergonomics, Ohio State University, cautions that to examine error, the definition of error must be clear. He suggests keeping track of three different senses of error:[18]

1. When you are talking about consequences: Consequence might be an injured patient or an extended length of stay.
2. When you are talking about hypothesized causes: Possible cause may be the checking system used to verify the correct bag of blood to be hung and infused.
3. When you are talking about deviation from standard: Deviation may be the variance in the sequence of fluid administration from accepted protocol.

Health care has largely focused on the adverse event as a consequence, limiting our knowledge of factors causing error through our limited attention to "near misses."

RESEARCH INTO ERROR AND ACCIDENT

Over the years, health care has focused on identifying the person responsible for the error and exacting some form of negative sanction or punishment. People are the problem. Other industries, such as the aviation industry, have found identifying "guilty" people to be an ineffective method for improving quality. These industries have found that looking at error as a systems failure, including systems of team function and communication, not failure of individual human beings, has been vastly more effective in improving quality.[19]

Health care organizations need to step back to objectively study the systems that surround the delivery of care by providers to patients to determine is what is required.

Researchers examining accidents have found a rich and illustrative story behind these judgments of human error. Going beyond the label of human error has helped pinpoint how complex systems fail. This understanding can lead to system improvement and prevention of errors. Human error should be a *starting* point for investigation, not the stopping point in a quality-driven organization.[20]

MODEL FOR THINKING ABOUT ERROR

The "Swiss-cheese" map (figure 3-2) illustrates that accidents or errors do not result from one single factor. Each factor is necessary to contribute to accidents in a complex system, and they are jointly sufficient to produce accidents. These factors are called latent errors. Using the logic of this model, attention is focused systemically on events and conditions that produce either a trajectory for error or a vulnerability for error.

In a health care setting, the confusion between similarly packaged medications may be identified by an attentive staff member or there might be systems that distinguish one medication from another through unit dose packaging. The inquiry becomes one of understanding the process flow rather than focusing on the practi-

FIGURE 3-2. Examples of Latent Errors

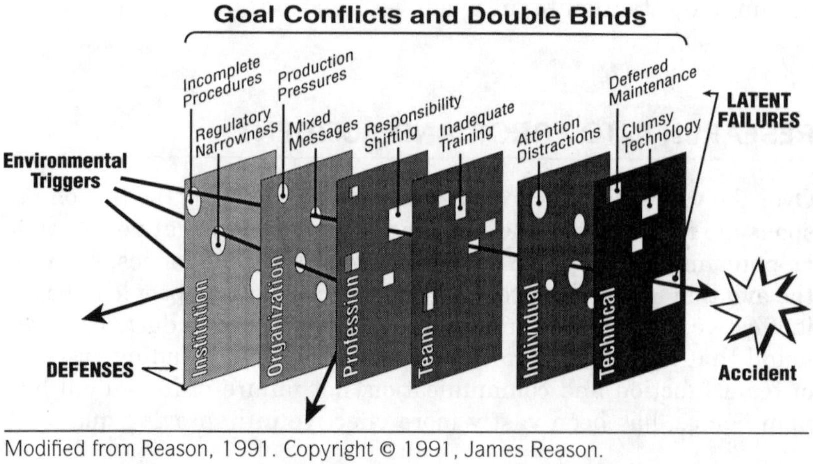

Modified from Reason, 1991. Copyright © 1991, James Reason.

tioner, who is the common pathway for the error experience.[21] The experience point of the error may be the provider, but the error is funneled by broad organizational, cultural, and systems issues, each contributing to the event.[22] Figure 3-3 illustrates the "blunt end" of the conditions, constituting the factors that can contribute to error: organization policies, procedures, and systems that are part of the environment in which providers and patients interact. These conditions directly affect the experience at the point of care—"the sharp end."

Health care has a higher degree of "surprise-factor" than other industries because we deal with human beings—their emotions and

FIGURE 3-3. Conditions That Directly Affect the "Sharp End"

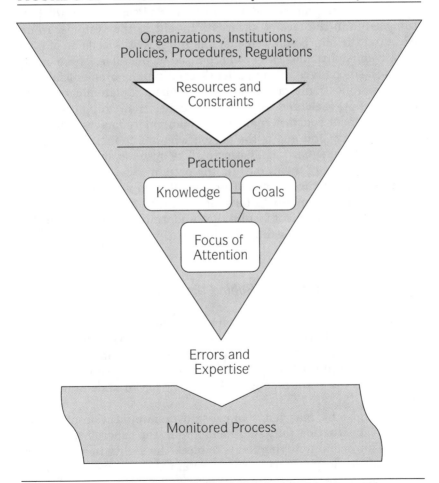

Reprinted, with permission, from: D. D. Woods, R. I. Cook, L. Johannsen, and N. Sorter, *Behind Human Error* (Hillside, NJ: Lawrence Erbaum, in press, 1998).

often unstable physiologic responses. Even so, there are considerable lessons to be learned from other industries and research.

Appreciating the Role of People on the "Sharp End"

In highly complex systems, such as a health care organization, people recognize that hazards exist and then design defenses against them. When defenses break down, latent failures come together to produce error. An important part of creating a safer environment is for people to recognize latent failures and redirect the trajectory away from accidents or adverse events.

The more figure 3-3 is examined, the more the experience of the provider at the sharp end is appreciated. People work to make things safe in the face of hazards inherent in the systems. To understand the sharp end, consider the nurse at the bedside of a patient who is physiologically compromised or unstable. There can be unexpected changes in the patient's condition, equipment failures, miscommunications, gaps in knowledge about a plan of care, variations in approach and skills of colleagues, new supplies due to product-vendor contract change, and many more factors. The nurse is at the sharp end and is the person who has to manage all these variables to safeguard against error. The systems, or lack of them, affect the safety of the nurse and the patient.

Focusing on the science of process flow and safety allows the identification of complex factors that can lead to error-prone situations and the removal of factors that undermine the provider's ability to safely and successfully provide care.

Understanding the Story Behind the Error

Counting errors and error rates may help focus on the issues needing attention. However, simple metrics cannot provide understanding. Behind and surrounding each error is the story about what happened. Successful methods of improvement are those that capture the story of the event and pursue the story for an understanding of the error.

In hindsight, bias tends to cause oversimplification of the details of the situation that staff members in the experience actually faced. This oversimplifying tends to block the ability to see and understand the deeper story.[23-25] Understandably, adverse events and errors challenge the fundamental beliefs about the safety of a system and demand explanation. In an attempt to explain what happened, people can isolate one factor from many contributing factors and label it "cause."

Errors will not be reduced until we replace reaction to error with scientific investigation of error using the tools and methods of quality improvement to eliminate root cause.

LESSONS FROM OTHER INDUSTRIES

Paul O'Neill, the CEO of Alcoa, gained the attention of industry when he declared that safety will be the number one priority of the company.[26] He focused on safety but hung other agendas on it, such as cost and productivity. If a worker fell off a machine, he asked: "What was he doing on the machine anyway? Was the machine designed with control mechanisms that actually increased risk?"

This is an example of leadership's explicit focus on the basics of safety. O'Neill recognized that safety could be a rallying focus for the workforce. By focusing on safety and pursuing the root causes of accidents, the company focused on improving process flow, which lead to increased productivity and reduced cost of error.

The aviation industry has focused relentlessly on the science of error reduction. There are some known actions, described by John Nance, that reduce the probability of error.[27] They are as follows:

- Simplify and standardize work processes and products such as the use of a consistent monitoring system.
- Design self-correcting systems or redundant systems that make it difficult to do the wrong thing, such as verifying messages about who will take what action when or using technical monitors to complement judgment.
- Reduce reliance on human memory through protocols, checklists, and automated systems.
- Use automation carefully through the meticulous design of manual processes that can be converted well to automation, such as the medication record documentation process.
- Learn how the function/organization works from studying it as a flow process. This requires a comprehensive audit of each step in a sequence.
- Drive out fear and set up systems so that data can be collected to learn about error and near misses. The risk should be in failing to report, not in the act of bringing bad news.
- Find out what is going on. Develop sources, ask questions. This is accomplished by being visible and actually reviewing in person the work activity.

- Do the obvious things one by one. When processes need correction, take action.

In pursuing the lessons in aviation, the value of making implicit knowledge explicit is essential. Implicit knowledge is the information and know-how that individuals uniquely possess. In health care, a great deal of the work in developing care paths or clinical pathways or best-of-practice models is about making explicit each provider's knowledge about how a care process works. Working to define the knowledge that people have and don't know they have is a critical step in understanding work flow and seeing the whole picture. It also helps focus on the question: *Who in the system has knowledge and who gets to ask the questions?*

The aviation industry would suggest that everyone has knowledge about different things and everyone can ask questions.[28] An illustration of the importance of shared knowledge and questioning is the example of the naval aircraft carrier flight deck, described in the article "When Failure Is Not an Option," by Robert Pool.[29] Berkeley researchers ask you to imagine the following:

Shrink your airport to only one short runway and one ramp and gate. Make planes take off and land at the same time, at half the present time interval, rock the runway from side to side, and require everybody to leave in the morning and return the same day. Turn off the radar to avoid detection, impose strict controls on radios, fuel the aircraft in place with their engines running, wet the whole thing down with salt water and oil, and man it with 20-year-olds, half who have never seen a plane close up.

This is not an exaggeration of the operating conditions of the Nimitz-class carriers. It is a remarkable story of the characteristics of an organization that is highly reliable in their ability to avoid error.

How can that organization operate so reliably? There are command, rules, and manuals of operating procedures that govern the flight deck process, making explicit lessons learned from years of experience. Navy training is designed to make these procedures second nature to the individuals who serve. But, as Berkeley researchers discovered, there is another dimension to this highly structured hierarchical organization.[30]

As pressure and risk mount during the launch and recovery of planes, the organizational structure shifts. Crew interact as colleagues, not superiors and subordinates. Cooperation and continual communication is part of the operation. With planes taking off and landing once a minute, things happen too quickly for instruction, delegation, and authorization to act. The crew works as a team by watching each other and by communicating constantly and repeatedly. The constant flow of observation and communication flags mistakes—the latent errors before they have caused damage (an accident/adverse event). Experienced personnel continually monitor the flow, listening for anything that doesn't fit and correcting mistakes before they cause error.

In an emergency, such as a deck fire, a third organizational structure emerges. If an emergency occurs, the crew reacts immediately and without direction. Each crew member assumes a preassigned role and fulfills the role according to carefully rehearsed procedures.

Here the welfare of the ship and crew is everyone's responsibility. Even the lowest ranking crew member has not only the authority but the obligation to suspend flight operations immediately under proper circumstances. "Although his judgment may later be reviewed or even criticized, he will not be penalized for being wrong and will often be publicly congratulated if right."[31]

LESSONS LEARNED FROM OTHER INDUSTRY APPLIED TO HEALTH CARE

As shown in the preceding aviation example, the involvement of everyone, combined with a healthy turnover of officers and crew, keeps people challenging old methods, learning new skills, and teaching them to others. The tension of bringing together fresh, even naive approaches with approaches that are built from years of history and experience, keeps safety and reliability a conscious, heedful set of actions rather than a mechanical repetition of following the rules. Think now about the clinic, the operating suite, the birthing center, the diagnostic laboratories, and how they operate. Most likely communication and actions are occurring against a gradient of hierarchy and in fear of negative sanctions.

Characteristics of High-Reliability Organizations

One large health care system engaged an expert author, speaker, and practitioner on airline safety to work with anesthesia-surgical teams in their operating room and perioperative care sites. The multidisciplinary teams engaged in lessons from the cockpit and the applications to their practice. Each team member developed an overall understanding of how the procedure unfolded and communicated any concerns that emerged. Staff members also learned to be wary of automated systems. Electronic systems have not provided the safety so many people have envisioned, so a high level of vigilance and judgment is required.[32]

High-reliability organizations are both centralized and decentralized, hierarchical and collegial, rule-bound and learning-centered. They also emphasize constant communication, even somewhat excessive communication, directed toward the purpose of avoiding mistakes. Constant watching and interacting is used to advise, detect, and act on any sign of trouble. In addition, high-reliability organizations look for ways to constantly improve and never take success or safety for granted. [33]

Common Factors in Safety

After extensive analysis of cases of failed safety, including the Exxon Valdez oil spill, the Chernobyl Soviet nuclear plant explosion, the Hubbel Telescope misguided mirror, and the Bhopal chemical gas spill in India, researchers Carolyn B. Libuser and Karlene Roberts have identified common factors in safety.[34]

Process Auditing   Process auditing involves establishing a system for ongoing checks and formal audits to spot unexpected safety problems. Questions for health care leaders include the following:

- Is there an internal audit function?
- Are key performance indicators systematically measured, reported, and reviewed?
- Is the quality function empowered to inquire, review, and measure critical areas of performance for the organization?
- Is a formalized framework for self-assessment used, such as the Baldrige criteria?
- Are accrediting surveys used as an opportunity for rigorous self-assessment?

Reward Systems   Are reward systems aligned consistently with promoting safe practice/behavior? The areas to focus on most critically are the cost-reduction pressures and mandates that most health care organizations are under. Are shortcuts being made to reduce costs? How are reward systems used to drive the attention and behavior of the organization? How is disclosure of risk- and failure-prone practices managed?

Pursual of Quality Standards   In the examples studied, standards for quality were subordinated to cost. Standards were not met for basic safety and industry standards. The issue is to monitor performance against industry best-in-class standards and to achieve that performance.

Perception of Risk   Perception of risk has two aspects: whether the organization or its members are aware of risks that exist, and if awareness of risk exists, what measures are being taken to minimize it? This relates to what data are collected, monitored, and acted on. In high-reliability organizations, there are effective monitoring systems and the organization acknowledges and confronts existing reality.

Command and Control   Formal rules and procedures are necessary. The issue here is adherence to the shared experience of best practice. This implies intelligent and thoughtful application of rules and procedures and not routinized ritual compliance. This factor is expanded by Roberts and Libuser, who outline command and control elements:[35]

- *Migrating decision-making:* The person with the most expertise makes the decision.
- *Having redundancy:* Back-up systems are in place, whether people or hardware exists.
- *Seeing the "big picture":* Senior managers see the big picture, and therefore do not micromanage, but attend to patterns and systems.
- *Establishing formal rules and procedures:* There is hierarchy and procedure/protocol based on evidence. This is not to be confused with bureaucracy.
- *Training:* Investment is made in the knowledge and skills of workers at the front line.

The researchers take each of the examples studied and analyze the failures against these characteristics of high-reliability organizations. A self-assessment against these criteria of characteristics of high-reliability organizations is a helpful step in determining the status of an organization and provides a baseline for action.

Health care leaders must determine whether there is ongoing rigorous assessment in place to continually understand the status of safety in their organizations. This is a different process than investigating errors and failures after they occur.

CONCLUSION

Health care is an industry in which new technology and techniques are introduced with exuberant fanfare. Failures are discarded in shadow. Failure in health care often disappears into bureaucratic and legal systems. Therefore, we know less about the topic of failure or error than do other industries. The complexity and interdependency within health care delivery and financing require that we become better informed, more aware, and take action to ensure that we are managing the basics. Safety, once taken for granted, takes vigilance, investment, and purposeful action to achieve.

Where can you start? Consider the following list promulgated by Dr. Donald Berwick:[36]

- Produce an economic analysis of the cost of an error in your organization.
- Investigate an adverse event. Personally interview the persons involved, reconstruct the pathway to the event, get coaching on the effects of hindsight bias.
- Invite a human factors consultant to observe a patient care unit or a patient care process and report back on compliance to the basics.
- Videotape one high-risk process for one-half hour. Send the tape to an expert to critique from a process flow perspective.

All providers depend on systems to deliver care, from local systems in a private office to complex systems in hospitals and communities, to the enormous systems of national health care. Instead of being victim to these systems and vulnerable for error, physicians, nurses, and health care managers can improve the system. Those who decide to abandon the search for bad apples, the defensive reaction to error, or what Berwick calls,[37] "the naiveté of an empty search for improvement through inspection and discipline" can study and apply the science of improvement to doing the basics consistently and reliably each and every time.

For safety and reduction of accidents and errors to be business imperatives of the organization, it will require a confidence and commitment by the leaders. Leaders will require managerial practices that examine the systemic nature of accidents and errors by assessing process flow. New expertise may be required so that performance is a feature of how processes and systems are designed. This means not only developing reliable team function but developing the science of understanding systems and process flow.

References

1. Nightingale, F., *Notes on Hospitals* (London, England: Longman, Green, Longman, Roberts, and Green, 1863).

2. Norman, D., *The Psychology of Everyday Things* (USA: Basic Books, a Division of Harper Collins, 1988).

3. Norman, p. 54.

4. Brennan, T. A., et al., "Incidence of Adverse Events and Negligence in Hospitalized Patients: Results from the Harvard Medical Practice Study I," *New England Journal of Medicine* 324 (1991): 370–6.

5. Leape, L. L., et al., "The Nature of Adverse Events in Hospitalized Patients: Results from the Harvard Medical Practice Study II," *New England Journal of Medicine* 324 (1991): 377–84.

6. Bates, D. W., et al., "Incidence of Adverse Drug Events and Potential Adverse Drug Events," *JAMA* 274, no. 1 (July 5, 1995).

7. Bootman, J. L., "The Health Care Cost of Drug-Related Morbidity and Mortality in Nursing Facilities," *Archives of Internal Medicine* 157 (Oct., 1997): 2089–96.

8. Johnson, J. A., and J. L. Bootman, "Drug-related Morbidity and Mortality and the Economic Impact of Pharmaceutical Care," *American Journal Health-System Pharmacy* 54 (Mar. 1, 1997).

9. Leape L. L., et al., "Preventing Medical Injury," *Quality Review Bulletin* (May, 1993): 144–9.

10. Leape, et al., *Quality Review Bulletin*, 1993.

11. Leape, et al., *Quality Review Bulletin*, 1993.

12. Leape, et al., *Quality Review Bulletin*, 1993.

13. Leape, et al., *Quality Review Bulletin*, 1993.

14. Leape, et al., *Quality Review Bulletin*, 1993.

15. Brennan, pp. 370–6.

16. Leape, et al., *Quality Review Bulletin*, 1993.

17. Leape, et al., *Quality Review Bulletin*, 1993.

18. Woods, D., Professor, Industrial and Systems Engineering, Ohio State University, Columbus, Ohio.

19. Helmreick, R., "Managing Human Error in Aviation," *Scientific American* (May, 1977): 62–7.

20. Woods, D., and R. Cook, excerpts from *Behind Human Error: Learning Systems Fail*, to be published by Lawrence Erlbaum, 1998.

21. Reason, J., *Human Error* (Cambridge, United Kingdom: Cambridge University Press, 1990): 208.

22. Cook, R., and D. Woods, *Working at the Sharp End: Achieving Patient Safety through Research*, a working paper, 1997.

23. Fischoff, 1975.

24. Fischoff, 1982.

25. Caplan, R. A., et al., "Adverse Anesthetic Outcomes arising from Gas Delivery Equipment: A Closed Claims Analysis," *Anesthesiology* 87, no. 4 (Oct. 1997): 741–8.

26. Smith, S. L., "Championing Compensation Costs in 1998," *Occupational Hazards* (December 1997): 30. Conversation with Robert A. Frosch, PhD, Senior Research Fellow, Belfer Center for Science and International Affairs, John F. Kennedy School of Government, Harvard University, Cambridge, Mass.

27. Nance, J. D., pilot/writer/author/consultant, board member, National Patient Safety Foundation and ABC News Analyst.

28. Pool, R., "When Failure Is Not an Option," *Microsoft Internet Explorer* (July, 1987): 1–6.

29. Pool, pp. 1–6.

30. Pool, pp. 1–6.

31. Pool, pp. 1–6.

32. Helmreick, pp. 62–7.

33. Pool, pp. 1–6.

34. Libuser, C. B., and K. Roberts, "Risk Mitigation through Organizational Structure," paper to be submitted, 1998.

35. Libuser and Roberts.

36. Berwick, D. (MD, MPP), President and CEO, Institute for Health Care Improvement, Recommendations to CEOs on Medical Error and Patient Safety.

37. Berwick, D., "Sounding Board—Continuous Improvement as an Ideal in Health Care," *The New England Journal of Medicine* 320, no. 1 (Jan. 5, 1989): 56.

Suggested Readings

ASHP Guidelines in Preventing Medication Errors in Hospitals, *American Journal of Hospital Pharmacy* 50 (Feb., 1993): 305–14.

ASHP Reports, "Suggested Definitions and Relationships Among Medication Misadventures, Medication Errors, Adverse Drug Events, and Adverse Drug Reactions," *American Journal Health-System Pharmacy* 55 (Jan. 15, 1998): 165–6.

Atman, C. J., et al., "Designing Risk Communications: Completing and Correcting Mental Models of Hazardous Processes, Part I," *Risk Analysis* 14, no. 5 (Oct., 1994): 779–88.

Bates, D. W., et al., "Incidents of Adverse Drug Events and Potential Adverse Drug Events," *JAMA* 274, no. 1 (July 5, 1995): 29–34.

Bates, D. W., et al., "The Costs of Adverse Drug Events in Hospitalized Patients," *JAMA* 277, no. 4 (Jan. 22/29, 1997): 307–11.

Bernstein, P. L., *Against the Gods: The Remarkable Story of Risk* (New York: John Wiley and Sons, 1996).

Berwick, D., "Quality Comes Home," *Quality Connection* 4, no. 1 (Winter, 1995): 1–4.

Bootman, J. L., "The Health Care Cost of Drug-Related Morbidity and Mortality in Nursing Facilities," *Archives of Internal Medicine* 157 (Oct. 13, 1997): 2089–96.

Bostrom, A., et al., "Designing Risk Communications: Completing and Correcting Mental Models of Hazardous Processes, Part I," *Risk Analysis* 14, no. 5 (Oct., 1994): 779–88.

Bostrom, A., et al., "Evaluating Risk Communications: Completing and Correcting Mental Models of Hazardous Processes, Part II," *Risk Analysis* 14, no. 5 (Oct., 1994): 789–98.

Caplan, R. A., et al., "Adverse Anesthetic Outcomes Arising from Gas Delivery Equipment: A Closed Claims Analysis," *Anesthesiology* 87, no. 4 (Oct., 1997): 741–8.

Classen, D. D., et al., "Computerized Surveillance of Adverse Drug Events in Hospital Patients," *JAMA* 266, no. 20 (Nov. 27, 1991): 2847–51.

Cullen, D., et al., "The Incident Reporting System Does Not Detect Adverse Drug Events: A Problem for Quality Improvement," Journal of Quality Improvement, *JCAHO* 21, no. 10 (1995): 541–8.

Eddy, D. M., "Guidelines for Policy Statements: The Explicit Approach," *Journal of the American Medical Association* 263, no. 16 (Apr. 25, 1990): 2239–40.

Hirschhorn, L., *Reworking Authority: Leading and Following in the Post-Modern Organization* (MIT Press: Cambridge, Mass., 1997).

Koch, B., "Differentiating Reliability Seeking Organizations from Other Organizations: Development and Validations of Assessment Devise."

Leape, L., et al. "Systems Analysis of Adverse Drug Events," *JAMA* 274, no. 1 (July 5, 1995): 35–43.

Lesar, T., et al., "Medication Prescribing Errors in a Teaching Hospital," *JAMA* 263, no. 17 (May 22, 1990): 2329–34.

National Patient Safety Foundation, for additional references, contact Web site http://www.ama-assn.org/med-sci/npsf/bibliogr.htm

Simms, M., *Wainwright Industries Safety—A Basic Human Need* (Cleveland: Penton Publishing, 1995.)

Smith, S. L., "How a Baldrige Winner Manages Safety," *Occupational Hazards* 57, no. 2 (Feb., 1995): 33.

Top-priority actions for preventing adverse drug events in hospitals. Recommendations of an expert panel. *American Journal Health-System Pharmacy* 53 (Apr. 1, 996): 47–51.

Understanding and Preventing Drug Misadventures. Published proceedings of a multidisciplinary invitational conference sponsored by the ASHP Research and Education Foundation in cooperation with AMA, ANA, ASHP, October 21–23, 1994, Chantilly, Va.

Weick, K. E., "Collective Mind in Organizations: Heedful Interrelating on Flight Decks," *Cornell University Graduate School of Business: Administrative Science Quarterly* 38, no. 3 (Sept., 1993): 357.

Weick, K. E., South Canyon Revisited: Lessons from High Reliability Organizations, Wildfire, December, 1955.

Weick, K., "Organizational Culture as a Source of High Reliability," *California Management Review* 29, no. 2 (Winter, 1987): 112–27.

Weick, K., "The Collapse of Sensemaking in Organizations: The Mann Gulch Disaster," *Cornell University Graduate School of Business: Administrative Science Quarterly* 38, no. 4 (Dec., 1993): 628.

4

Building a Practical Quality Model

To understand and improve work, it is necessary to make work explicit. This means to clearly identify assumptions about how things happen and relate to one another to produce results. Models allow the organization to be explicit about how work is organized and done, to explore the interdependencies and dynamic complexities of differing parts of an organization that do work, and to measure the results or effects of work. Applying gauges or measures to parts of a model allows us to promote processes for improvement in all dimensions of work.

The dictionary defines *model* as a miniature representation of something, a structural design or set of plans for building, an example for emulation. A model is also used to help others visualize something that cannot be directly observed; for example, a model may be designed for a system or state of affairs so that calculations and predictions can be made.[1] Implementation of quality roles and responsibilities occurs within a context of how the organization operates. A model is a depiction of how things work. The organizational model is a way of understanding how the organization operates and how the parts of the organization relate to and affect each other.

This chapter presents three examples of how to build a practical model for quality that has relevance to understanding how the organization can operate: a quality-driven organizational model, a value chain model, and a patient care delivery model.

QUALITY-DRIVEN ORGANIZATIONAL MODEL

Historically, quality has been assigned to a department of specialized staff or a quality officer who is engaged to meet accreditation and regulatory compliance or to pursue excellence in times of favorable financial performance. This function was often appended to an organizational chart. Suspend that model of quality. Instead, imagine quality in this way:

> Quality is a value and a discipline of knowledge, skills and practices to achieve excellence in products, service and environment based on the requirements, perceptions and future needs of our customer.[2]

Quality now becomes how an organization does its work. Quality principles and practices are a part of how each member of the organization understands and implements his or her role.

Imagine an organization that is clear about its priorities and focus, has decision-making processes in place, and is grounded in the use of data and statistical thinking to intelligently create and guide change. Imagine further that desired results are articulated and measurements are used to determine progress to achieve the results. Most important, imagine this organization is steeped in customer knowledge and totally driven by the customer needs and preferences in products, care, and services. The workforce is prepared and strives to exceed customer requirements, continually challenging and improving its work. This is the culture of quality that demonstrates best-of-practice in clinical care, leads the competition in service excellence, has a committed and competent workforce, and has a track record of effective strategy execution and cost reduction through elimination of waste and the costs of poor quality. It leads the market in customer loyalty.

The model shown in figure 4-1 is based on the Malcolm Baldrige criteria and provides the framework to build a quality-driven organization designed for performance and results. The model is divided into three dimensions: driver, system, and results. Leadership is the engine that drives this model by building integrated systems. These systems are designed to acquire customer knowledge, engage in strategic quality planning, develop human resources, and manage the processes of an organization. Figure 4-2 (p. 74) outlines the Baldrige criteria that comprise this quality-driven model. These categories and items are divided according to the three dimensions depicted in the model: driver (leadership), system (integrated work processes), and results (financial, clinical, loyalty).

FIGURE 4-1. Model for a Quality-Driven Organization

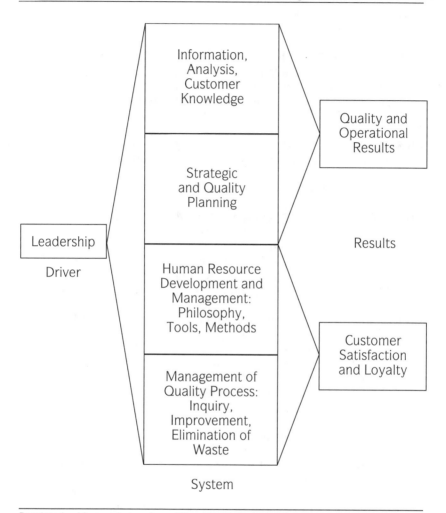

Reprinted, with permission, from Allina Health System, Minnetonka, Minn., 1998.

Driver

De Hock, the founder of VISA, is quoted to have said, "A commercial company, or for that matter any organization, is nothing but a mental construction, a concept, an idea to which people are drawn in pursuit of common purpose."[3] Leadership through vision and example inspires a deep sense of purpose. The Wharton School started its first leadership course for executives in the late 1980s, about the

FIGURE 4-2. 1992 Baldrige Criteria

Categories & Items	Maximum Points
1.0 Leadership	**90**
1.1 Senior Executive Leadership	45
1.2 Management for Quality	25
1.3 Public Responsibility	20
2.0 Information & Analysis	**80**
2.1 Scope and Management of Quality, Performance Data, and Information	15
2.2 Competitive Comparisons and Benchmarks	25
2.3 Analysis of Uses of Company-Level Data	40
3.0 Strategic Quality Planning	**60**
3.1 Strategic Quality and Company Performance Planning Process	35
3.2 Quality and Performance Plans	25
4.0 Human Resource Development & Management	**150**
4.1 Human Resource Management	20
4.2 Employee Involvement	40
4.3 Employee Education and Training	40
4.4 Employee Performance and Recognition	25
4.5 Employee Well-Being and Morale	25
5.0 Management of Process Quality	**140**
5.1 Design and Introduction of Quality Products and Services	40
5.2 Process Management–Product, Service Production, and Delivery Processes	35
5.3 Process Management–Business Process and Support Services	30
5.4 Supplier Quality	20
5.5 Quality Assessment	15
6.0 Quality & Operational Results	**180**
6.1 Product and Service Quality Results	75
6.2 Company Operational Results	45
6.3 Business Process and Support Service Results	25
6.4 Supplier Quality Results	35
7.0 Customer Focus & Satisfaction	**300**
7.1 Customer Relationship Management	65
7.2 Commitment to Customers	15
7.3 Customer Satisfaction Determination	35
7.4 Customer Satisfaction Results	75
7.5 Customer Satisfaction Comparisons	75
7.6 Future Requirements and Expectations of Customers	35

Reprinted, with permission, from George, Stephen, *The Baldrige Quality System* (John Wiley & Sons, 1992).

time those in business realized the vast organizational, societal, and marketplace changes they faced and became aware of the need for a new kind of leadership.[4]

However, mere leadership command and control were not sufficient in confronting the need to improve quality. Early efforts at total quality, announced as a top-down campaign, failed. Quality improvement was more than introducing new tools and methods. It included a new way of leading and managing that required the personal commitment of leaders and the redistribution of power, purpose, and wealth.[5] Leaders provided clear directions and detailed objectives so that the quality challenges could be identified and met.

In *Driving Change*, Wind and Main cite leaders such as Bob Gavin of Motorola and Jamie Houghton of Corning as exemplars who reinvented leadership to embed quality in their organizations.[6] The same chapter on leadership more fully explores the leader's role in developing shared vision and values, commitment to purpose, clarity about focus, and quality as a performance imperative that characterized the leadership of Gavin and Houghton.

Leaders, such as Jack Welch of General Electric, clearly state that an effort to improve quality would be "the most personally rewarding and, in the end, most profitable undertaking in our history."[7] Developing leaders is a serious and deliberate undertaking at General Electric. More than 30 percent of Welch's time is committed to developing leaders. Using the metaphor of the driver, Welch is reported to have one instrument by which he drives the quality of the company—the accelerator.

System

For purposes of simplicity, the model breaks the system or operations of the organization into four dimensions: information, analysis, and customer knowledge; strategic and quality planning; human resource development and management; and management of quality process.

Entire books could be dedicated to the examination of each system dimension. This chapter briefly describes each dimension and its quality function, inviting the reader to pursue the subject in greater depth.

Information, Analysis, and Customer Knowledge   A quality-driven organization is managed by fact, not opinion, and needs information to support evidence-based decision making and to gauge improvement. Information is a key resource that must be available to people throughout the organization. Profound understanding of the customer is the foundation for strategic planning, and customer feedback is the basis for evaluating the results of the company's work. Although advanced information system technology is ideal for data repository, access to data, and ease of dissemination of data, much can be learned by talking to the customer in a systematic way, using simple methods to collect data, and communicating to the organization what has been learned. The message here is not to wait until the state-of-the-art information system is installed. Start now and be diligent about acquiring customer information.

The following specific actions need to be taken:

- Link customer knowledge to strategic planning and action plan development.
- Increase information sharing and coordination of efforts (establish advisory bodies for customer groups: employees, physicians, patients, members, employer purchasers).
- Incorporate customer requirements in surveys with coordination of survey administration and trending of results.
- Create a customer knowledge database by pooling sources of information, such as market research, satisfaction surveys, focus groups, complaint information, and other methods to listen to customers.
- Develop training modules (selection of methods, collection processes, interpretation, application of results) that emphasize listening skills for management, staff, and physicians.
- Increase employees' customer contact time (even for those not typically in contact roles).
- Develop a module on customer information for employee orientation.
- Revise job descriptions to reflect that gaining and using customer knowledge are part of the job.
- Involve customers in redesign and improvement efforts.
- Invest in expertise (statistician, survey analysts) to help interpret and use customer data for improvement.

Strategic and Quality Planning A strategic plan is not complete unless it includes quality, program and financial considerations, and a clear pathway to reach the organization's vision. A quality-driven organization designs its planning process around a customer and market focus to ensure that the following content areas are explicitly addressed:

- Customer knowledge
- Competitive quality performance
- Product and service performance

- Reduction in deficiencies
- Improvement of macro processes
- Costs of poor quality

In addition to content, the planning process will have the following characteristics:

- Physician involvement
- Stakeholder involvement
- Interactive and engaging development
- Action driven by customer requirements
- The basis for financial/resource requirements
- Systemic perspective
- Cycle of evaluation for planning
- Prioritized and focused activities
- Highly communicated goals and strategies
- Well-detailed and measurable milestones

In the planning process itself, the Hoshin-Kanri process can help the organization determine where to focus its efforts to achieve breakthroughs of high performance.[8] The process involves "catchball," or tossing ideas up and down the organization, so that alignment of thinking is achieved. Hoshin planning and goal setting can also be used to disseminate information and to support strategy implementation. Figure 4-3 depicts the key elements of the process.

Human Resource Development and Management   The human resources function is a powerful instrument in creating a culture of quality. The culture of the organization is the embodiment of the organization's values and operating philosophy. It can be described as "the way we act here." The culture of the organization is expressed through the behavior of its employees and their day-to-day actions; the modes of communicating and decision making; and the policies, procedures, structures, and incentives being used. The congruence between "the way we act here" and what is espoused is critical. Alienation and cynicism develop in gaps that exist if there is not congruence. This is a critical issue for quality as a driving business strategy. Alignment of philosophy, policy, procedure, recognition, and incentives to the philosophy and principles of quality is essential. A careful assessment of this is an important and essential exercise. Areas to be reviewed include the following:

- Management philosophy and practices
- Investment in employee and leadership development of essential skills

FIGURE 4-3. Key Elements of the Hoshin Process

In the function of quality planning, Hoshin-Kanri is an approach to the development and execution of quality strategies to focus the efforts of Allina to achieve breakthroughs of high performance for customers. The Hoshin process is a method to align the organization to achieve results. Hoshin planning and goal setting is also a deployment technique for strategy implementation.

A brief description of the Hoshin process follows:

Hoshin Goals

Main Purpose	Organization problem solving for breakthroughs
Focus	Business capabilities in meeting/exceeding customer, consumer and stakeholder expectations and perceptions
Execution	Teams
Responsibility	Participation
Methodology	Quality principles, methods, tools
Time Horizon	Annual activity aligned with long-term goal
Review	Periodic progress on process and results
Objective Priority	Vital few for competitive advantage
Decision Basis	Facts and data
	Customer perspective

- Clearly articulated performance competencies, reflected in job descriptions and performance reviews, and opportunities for performance improvement
- Manager and employee expectations and evaluations based on contribution to quality
- Rewards and recognitions for contributions to quality
- Supplier selection and retention requirements
- Assessment of competitive quality performance: how do we monitor and react?
- Product and service development and performance requirements
- Customer communication (especially listening to the customer) and management of relationships with customers
- Employee participation in the quality process: who participates (and under what circumstances/conditions) and will

process improvement be mandated as part of all operating plans?

- Employee apprehension: how do we respond to questions about job security in the context of quality improvement?
- The labor-management philosophy, structure, and practices

Human resource processes are a powerful lever for change because the reinforcement of employees' behaviors creates positive change. Conversely, failure to achieve appropriate alignment can be costly and wasteful in the loss of commitment, energy, and contributions of the people in the organization.

Management of Quality Process As outlined in the preface to this book, there are leadership and managerial methods that advance quality. Measurement and infrastructure requirements also need to be in place for quality processes to be effective. These are discussed in chapters 6 and 9. When quality is identified as a strategic imperative, the process needs to have clear priorities, be aligned with the organization's goals, and be monitored continuously for results.

Results

The result of a well-integrated, well-managed quality model is performance excellence: favorable quality, operational results, and customer loyalty. The model helps the organization understand itself as a system; that is, a collection of interdependent people, processes, products, and services that are focused on and aligned with a common purpose.

The Baldrige Framework is helpful to use when thinking about functional organizational integration and alignment. Detailed examination of the Baldrige model, along with applications for self-assessment in each dimension, can be found in *The Baldrige Quality System*, authored by Stephen George.[9]

VALUE CHAIN MODEL

An adaptation of the Harvard Value Chain, this model helps make explicit the business logic of the organization.[10] Figure 4-4 shows how the model tracks employees' perspectives and attitudes about customer satisfaction, health improvement, and financial results.

FIGURE 4-4. Health System Employee-Customer-Results Chain

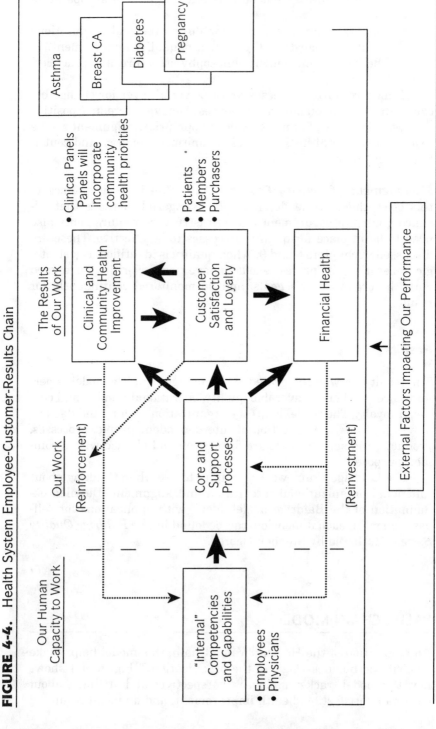

Reprinted, with permission, from Allina Health System, Minnetonka, Minn., 1998.

The Model's Measurement System

A measurement system is designed to gauge the performance of key factors in the model. The model and its underlying assumptions are tested by measures that gauge employees' perspectives of the work environment; services, products, or care based on customer key work processes; and results of work effort measured by customer satisfaction and loyalty, health improvement, and financial health.

By placing measures on the different parts of the model, it is possible to determine how the organization actually works. For example, a systematic surveying of employees' perspectives informs the organization of the human resource function as experienced by the employees. The measures test the model and inform an organization's members about the validity of the model. Because there is a model that stabilizes and documents beliefs and understandings about organizational functions and operations, learning can take place and predictions can be made about how a change in one part of an organization will affect another part.

The model's assumption is that committed employees who find their work meaningful will be better able to serve the customer. Prepared with customer knowledge, employees will produce valued products and provide services that delight the customer. This, in turn, will produce a satisfied and loyal customer, resulting in market share and the ability to influence health behavior over time. Opportunities to improve health outcomes and profits will be realized. Rigorous measurement actively tests these assumptions.

Subsequent chapters focus on the measurement systems required. However, in this chapter, it is important to note that without a model, measurement can be used neither as a strategic tool to examine the operations of the organization nor as a tool to manage improvement.

The measures used to test how the business operates are called the key performance indicators. The goal of the model's measurement system is to make predictions and anticipate change: When a change occurs in one part of the model, what change might be expected to occur in another part? For example, if the assumptions underlying the model are accurate, then a decline in employees' morale about the organization would affect its financial performance, although there may be a lag before finances are affected.

One Adaptation of the Model

Although the model depicted in figure 4-4 is relatively new to health care (1996),[11] Sears has been working on a parallel course fueled by devastating financial losses in 1992.[12] Then, a new CEO arrived and engineered an impressive turnaround. A detailing of this turnaround, published in the *Harvard Business Review*, describes the development of an employee-customer-profit chain model and the rigorous measures associated with it that helped them hold the gains and make further improvements.[13] Tools, training, and management practices were built around the model to focus the efforts of the company. The Sears model, shown in figure 4-5, illustrates the Harvard Value Chain as applied to a retail business.

As Sears has gained experience with this model, the company has been able to predict across space and time the degree to which changes in one part of the organization affect the other parts of the organization. This predictive power allows simulations and scenario building to test changes in theory before they become business reality.

PATIENT CARE DELIVERY MODEL

The final model, a patient care delivery model, is shown in figure 4-6 (p. 84). This model reflects delivery of care services, a part of health improvement. The same requirements of organizational models underlie the needs of a patient care delivery model. The patient care delivery model described in this chapter is the result of a two-year development and improvement process that reflected how care is delivered.[14] The purpose of this model is to present a stable view of the care process, understand it, and improve it. The model is a representation—on paper—of how care is actually delivered. Like organization models, measures that gauge customer satisfaction can be used to measure satisfaction with the process.

The measures applied to this model are the dimensions of care used in the Picker Patient Satisfaction Survey Instrument,[15] described in detail in chapter 2. The specific dimensions—access, emotional support, respect, patient and family involvement, information and education, and continuity and transition—measure the patient's experience with the delivery of care. Through measured performance within these dimensions, the organization can gauge its progress in providing patients with what they believe is important.

Assumptions underlying the patient care delivery model include the following:

- Care is patient-focused, with the patient actively participating in the care process.

FIGURE 4-5. Employee-Customer-Profit Chain at Sears

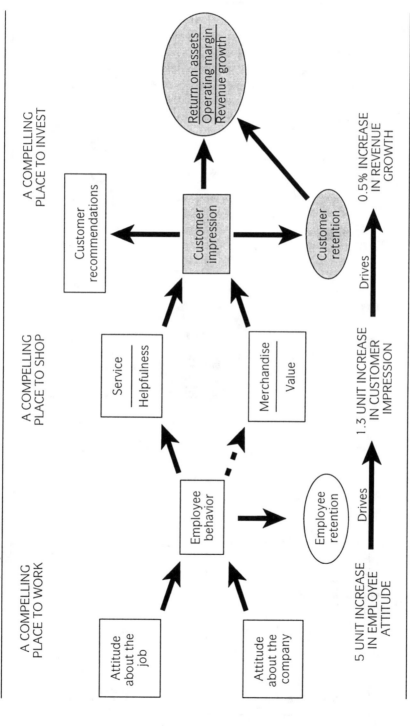

Reprinted by permission of *Harvard Business Review*. [An Exhibit]. From "The Employee-Customer-Profit Chain at Sears" by Anthony J. Rucci, Steven P. Kirn, and Richard T. Quinn (Jan.-Feb., 1998).

FIGURE 4-6. Patient Care Delivery Model

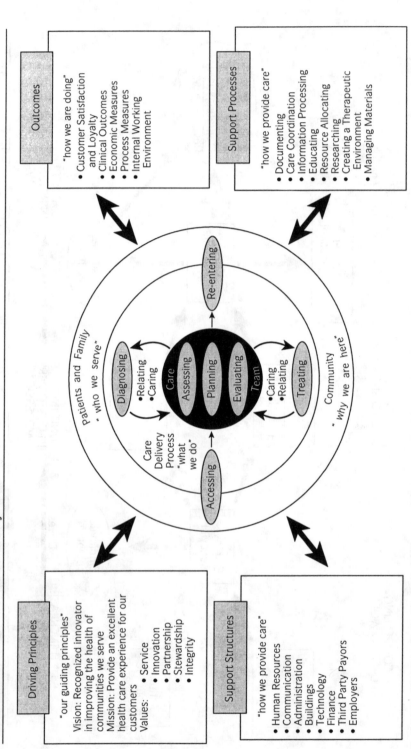

Reprinted, with permission, from Allina Health System, Minnetonka, Minn., 1998.

- All participants (patients, family, community, caregivers, support persons and payers) are included in care delivery.
- Health care professionals offer unique and shared services and are accountable and responsible for decisions about the health status of individuals served.
- Excellence in health care delivery results from an atmosphere of respect, interdisciplinary interaction, and cooperation. Care delivery and its improvement are team efforts.
- Care delivery occurs in a learning environment.
- Systems thinking (holistic and interactive) is essential.

Components of the Patient Care Delivery Model

Essential components in the patient care delivery model include the following:

- Customers (patients and families) and the communities to which they return
- Care delivery processes (accessing, assessing, diagnosing, planning, treating, evaluating, and re-entering)
- Driving principles
- Outcomes
- Support structures
- Support processes

Each of the components in patient care delivery is essential to comprehensive, quality care. It is important to emphasize that each component affects another; the arrows on the model show this interaction. All components, working together, are important to the delivery of patient care. The following describes each component of the model.

Customers   Customers encircle the care delivery processes because they are "who we serve" and "why we are here." The patient and family are who we serve. The entire episode of care, including ambulatory, inpatient, home care, and community-based care, are included in the delivery of care.

Care Delivery Processes   The care delivery process is the reason health care delivery exists; it is "what we do." It includes accessing; assessing; diagnosing; planning; treating; evaluating; and re-entering a hospital, home, or another care facility. Accessing is the process of acquiring the information, communicating with a knowledgeable provider, getting an appointment, or entering a care site.

Assessing and *diagnosing* include clinical (hands on), laboratory, radiologic, and other diagnostic processes. *Planning* includes strategic/quality plans and the patient/family plan of care. *Treating* includes drugs, procedures, counseling, teaching, and care in support of patient oxygenation, circulation, behavior, perception, mobility, nutrition, elimination, immunity, and parent/baby. *Re-entering* is the process of an informed patient moving to another level of care, site of care, agency, or provider relationship. Evaluating is the process used to determine whether interventions were effective and helpful to the patient and family served. It answers the question whether improvement in health occurred. Caring and relating pervade the care processes and are a holistic valuing of each patient and team member. They include a team approach, patient participation in decision making, ethics in each interpersonal interaction, communication techniques and vehicles, a value for diversity, and support for the interdependencies of roles. Relating is primary in the diagnostic phase; caring is primary in the treatment phase.

The use of *we* in the model implies that the team is essential to the patient care processes. "Who we are" includes the caregivers—physicians, nurses, pharmacists, dietitians, social workers, and staff from other disciplines who deliver their services near patient care. Also included are referring and consulting resources and community and other social and spiritual supports.

Driving Principles and Outcomes   Driving principles and outcomes are the visionary and marketplace forces that drive patient care. The driving principles of the model contain guiding principles. The vision, mission, and values are lived by all those providing care. The principles are patient-centered, quality-oriented, and cost-effective.

Outcomes are marketplace forces that describe "how we are doing." Outcomes are the results of care and include customer satisfaction and loyalty, clinical outcomes, economic measures, process measures, and an index of the internal working environment.

Support Structures and Support Processes   Support structures and support processes explain how care is provided and describe the elements that support care. The support structures are basic to care delivery and include buildings and their physical environment. Other support structures are human resources, marketing, administration, technology, finance, third-party payers, employers, and regulators such as the Joint Commission on Accreditation of Healthcare Organizations (Joint Commission) and National Committee on Quality Assurance (NCQA).

The support processes strengthen care, are accessible to the patient and team, and include the following:

- *Documentation:* Documentation includes written patient care and system information.
- *Care coordination:* Care coordination emphasizes coordination of care and information across providers and time.
- Information processing: Information processing includes data management and decision-support mechanisms.
- *Education:* Education includes use of teaching/learning principles and products for patients, team members, and students. Competency and credentialling of providers are vital aspects of education.
- *Resource allocation:* Resource allocation includes areas such as staffing, hiring, and purchasing.
- *Research:* Evaluation, research, and monitoring include daily patient evaluation, peer review, and retrospective and prospective studies. Processes such as improvement initiatives, utilization review, evaluation, research, and research utilization are also used.
- *Therapeutic environment:* A therapeutic environment is created by ensuring that the aspects of caring and relating exist and that a safe, clean, and welcome care delivery area exists.
- *Materials management:* Materials management is having cost-effective materials available in a timely manner at the point of care.

Application of the Patient Care Delivery Model

The Patient Care Delivery Model serves as the basis for understanding the care delivery system and for managing the improvement system. Its use spans departments, programs, services, distance (patient, home, community, and hospital), and time (the entire episode of care). The care delivery model focuses on the customer and the center of care and accurately describes the process of caring for patients. It enables those in all parts of the system to see their role in the process. The model supports integrated health care by encouraging dialogue and interaction across parts of the system, across disciplines, and across departments on behalf of the customer, emphasizing an interdependence that promotes comprehensive care. It provides a framework for managing improvement and measuring outcomes by creating a vehicle to study and stabilize the process of care so that improvement opportunities can be identified and action can be taken. The model strengthens planning by providing a structure for incorporating quality and operations considerations around the needs of customers and measures the organization's collective performance at delivering products and services. The model supports improvements in multidisciplinary clinical practice by making explicit the staff's assumptions about the care delivery process and the role of all disciplines who contribute to it.

CONCLUSION

The development of models provides a description of complex processes so that interrelationships and causal linkages can be studied. They allow us to be explicit about employees' assumptions of how things work. By being explicit, we can measure performance and test assumptions embedded in the model to see how things really *do* work. The power of models is that they provide the context for measures and the impetus for improvement. They also allow us to see, understand, and predict changes that may occur in one part of the system based on changes occurring in other parts.

To be successful, an organization must leave room to change the model, in case it is not the correct one. Measures will let you know whether a model is successful. However, a model is only a conceptual rendering. How to implement the model is explored in the following chapters. Will Rogers once said, "I'll give you a dollar for a model, and a million dollars for its implementation." The success of an organization is the right model, the ability to implement the model, and the ability to use it to drive positive change.

References

1. Allen, R. E., ed., *The Concise Oxford Dictionary of Current English,* 8th edition (Oxford: Clarendon Press, 1990): 762.

2. *The Quality Blueprint,* Allina Health System, Minnetonka, Minn., 1996.

3. Wind, J. Y., and J. Main, *Driving Change: How the Best Companies Are Preparing for the 21st Century* (New York: The Free Press, 1998): 94.

4. Wind and Main, p. 94.

5. Block P., Stewardship: *Choosing Service over Self-Interest* (San Francisco: Berrett-Koehler, 1993).

6. Wind and Main, p. 94.

7. Welch, J. W., Jr. (Chairman, General Electric Company), speech to the Annual Meeting of Stockholders, Charlottesville, Va., Apr. 24, 1996.

8. Melum, M. M., and C. Colett, *Breakthrough Leadership: Achieving Organizational Alignment through Hoshin Planning* (Chicago: American Hospital Publishing, 1995): 17.

9. George, S., *The Baldrige Quality System: The Do-It-Yourself Way to Transform Your Business* (New York: John Wiley and Sons, 1992).

10. Heskett, J. L., et al., "Putting the Service Profit Chain to Work," *Harvard Business Review* (Mar.-Apr., 1994).

11. Bushik, B., and J. Morath, Allina Health System, Minnetonka, Minn., 1996.

12. Rucci, A. J., S. P. Kirn, and R. Quinn, "The Employee-Customer-Profit Chain at Sears," *Harvard Business Review* 76(1) (Jan.-Feb., 1998): 83–97.

13. Rucci, Kirn, and Quinn, pp. 83–97.

14. Hogan-Miller, E., et al., Abbott Northwestern Hospital, Minneapolis, Minn., 1997.

15. Gerteis M., et al., *Through the Patient's Eyes* (San Francisco: Jossey-Bass Health Series, 1993): 19–40.

Suggested Readings

Heskett, J., W. E. Sasser, and L. Schlesinger, *The Service Profit Chain* (New York: Free Press, 1997).

Leonard, F. S., and W. E. Sasser, "The Incline of Quality," *Harvard Business Review* 60 (Sept., 1982): 163.

Normann, R., and R. Ramirez, "From Value Chain to Value Constellation: Designing Interactive Strategy," Comment in *Harvard Business Review* 5 (Sept.-Oct., 1993): 39–40, 42–3, 46–51.

5

Creating the Infrastructure for a Quality-Driven Organization

Whether leaders are on the front line or in the highest level of the company, the goal of a quality-driven organization is for all members of the organization to embody a passion to serve the customer and to have a hardiness for change, a loyalty to the truth, a willingness to inquire into better methods of performance, and an intolerance for waste. A quality organization does not simply happen. It takes time, leadership commitment, and consistent investment of resources over time. This is not a blitz initiative or campaign. Quality cannot be inserted into an organization. It must be carefully, skillfully, and persistently built inside the organization itself.

Like the infrastructure required to build a house—the foundation, support beams, wiring, heating and plumbing systems—an organization needs infrastructure to build the capacity for employees to learn and improve. These essential infrastructure elements must be part of the formal operating policies and procedures of the organization so that skills and practices are reinforced, rewarded, and sustained.

This chapter describes the elements of an organizational infrastructure that will enable people to continually improve their work. These elements include providing development and training opportunities; choosing the appropriate team sponsors and facilitators; and incorporating the processes, structures, and practices that will enable people to apply what they have learned toward realizing their improvement efforts.

PROVIDING DEVELOPMENT AND
TRAINING OPPORTUNITIES

The first necessary element of the organizational infrastructure is the process that enables people to continually improve their work—to eliminate waste, better serve customers, and make improvements. This process involves development and training techniques that put the knowledge and tools of improvement squarely in the hands of the providers and employees closest to the work.

The organization must provide a range of opportunities for all employees to learn and practice quality improvement. For this development and training to succeed, an organization must have the facilitators and consultants necessary to help teams as they advance their work.

Model for Employee Education and Quality Training

One approach to employee education and quality training can be depicted in a building block model (figure 5-1).[1] This model demonstrates the construction of knowledge from a foundational platform to increasingly complex layers of skills that are necessary for leadership roles. The building blocks or content areas for education and training are designed so that new information and more advanced skills are added as foundational content is integrated and applied in an individual's work. This model uses the work of Peter Senge in understanding a "learning organization"; that is, an organization in which staff members are constantly learning from the customer, understanding work from a process flow perspective, working in teams, and applying a discipline so that they can practice improvement constantly.[2] The *Fifth Discipline Fieldbook* offers a practical guide to understanding, applying, and nurturing these foundational skills.[3] Through development and training techniques, employees can develop an essential component of continuous improvement in organizations—the ability to work effectively in teams, to honor the contributions of each member, and to develop the collective spirit to perform together.

Health care is an industry that requires people-working teams to perform consistently and reliably. For staff in an emergency department, operating room, or intensive care unit, the ability to work in a coordinated effort is crucial to a patient's outcome. Yet, as described in chapter 3, health care is not as advanced as other indus-

FIGURE 5-1. Quality Education/Development Building Blocks

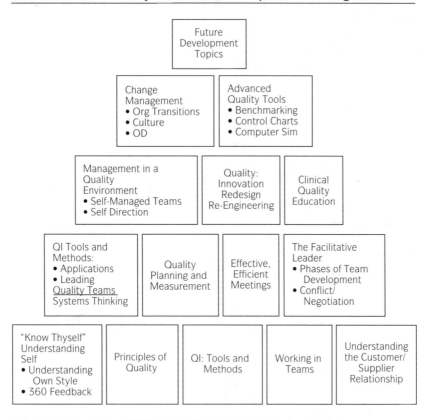

Reprinted, with permission, from Allina Health System, Minnetonka, Minn., 1998.

tries in the science and skills of teamwork. Training in teamwork is critical to improving health care quality.

Training provides the opportunity to clarify organizational expectations, identify roles and responsibilities, develop a common language, validate the understanding of values and principles that guide quality, legitimize the conversations that should take place around improvement, and create a safe place to test new knowledge and tools. Training also provides an opportunity for ongoing education and for staff members to be introduced to the infrastructure supports, educational services, and consultative resources the organization has.

FIGURE 5-1A. Quality Building Blocks

Programming Modules

A. Personal development
- Understand human dynamic
  - Learning
  - Communications
  - Conflict management
  - Conditions for stress
  - Affinities for function
  - Developmental direction
- Personal strengths and vulnerabilities
- Similarities and differences in leadership and followership
- Self-initiated 360 degree feedback
- Personal development planning

B. Working in teams
- Understanding self in relationship to others
- Team dynamics and development
- Conflict and collaboration
- Communicating for "shared meaning/shared understanding"
- Roles/responsibilities/accountabilities

C. Principles of quality
- The approach to quality
- Core organizational processes
- Change processes
- Structure and teams
- Common language
- Quality resources

Competency: Cultural knowledge

D. Change process 1: tools and methods
- The change process
- The roles and responsibilities of team members
- Skill-building for process improvement
  - Developing team charters
  - Brainstorming/motivating
  - Flowcharts and C-E diagrams
  - Pareto and histograms
  - Data collection and analysis
  - Cost benefit and force field analysis
  - Implementation, evaluating and monitoring plans

Competency: Process improvement

E. Customer/supplier relationships
- Customer as partner
- Analysis of customer needs/requirements
- Responsiveness
- Value chains
- Forging partnerships

Competency: Customer-focused

F. The facilitative leader
- Management versus leadership
- Influence versus power
- Vision and common goals
- Interactive communication
- Process facilitation

Competency: Team leadership

G. Effective, efficient meetings
- Roles and responsibilities
- Ground rules and norms
- Attending to agenda
- Evaluation and minutes
- Managing process

Competency: Productive meetings

H. The planning/development process
- Mission, vision, core processes, and strategic initiatives
- Shared customer requirements
- Program/departmental planning in the organizational context
- Critical success factors and targeted outcomes
- Departmental processes
- Measuring and monitoring outcomes

Competency: Organizational alignment

I. Change process 2: tools and methods application
- Application of process improvement tools and methods through case studies
- Systems thinking:
  - "Friday night at the emergency room"
  - Causal loop diagrams
  - Flight simulators

How to Begin Quality Improvement

As an infrastructure element, training is typically the most underestimated. It has been reported that Baldrige Quality Award recipients invest more than four percent of their total budgets to the development of the human capital of their organizations—the employees.

Focus on Real-Life Applications   To be effective, training must be focused on real-life applications or on real problems or issues. Thus, the content for any training in quality transfers the tools and methods of improvement squarely into the hands of the people doing the work. Training begins through the search for answers to the following fundamental questions:

- What are the vision, mission, and values of the organization? What is the philosophy or principles of quality for the organization?
- Who are the customers, and what do they need?
- What are the organization's resources to support quality improvement efforts?

Those involved in the training can begin to examine their environment in more detail by asking the following questions:

- How do we create and use tools such as cause-and-effect diagrams, force field analyses, control charts, chart interpretation, histograms, Pareto diagrams, and scatter diagrams to stabilize and understand our organization's systems?
- How do we approach and manage data collection, including formulating the question, choosing data and data sources, and conducting sampling and stratification?
- How do we use basic descriptive statistics to describe central tendency and spread or variability and to provide visual representation?
- How do we conduct cost-benefit analysis?
- How do we use implementation tools such as planning and implementation worksheets, tree diagrams, Gantt charts, and storyboards?

Through the use of quality tools, team members can also enrich their work by exploring the answers to the following questions:

- How do we develop team charters that include problem statements, goal statements, measures, parameters, members, ground rules, and functions for the team?
- How do we use decision-making tools such as consensus, brainstorming, multivoting, weighted voting, and decision matrices?
- How do we use flowcharts of process mapping, matrix or deployment flowcharts, high-level or detail flowcharts, top-down flowcharts, and layout flowcharts?

By including an introduction to quality tools and their specific purpose, the training provides individuals with an opportunity to match the tool to the task and use the tool effectively.

Initiate Just-in-Time Timing Training that is distant in time to its application is training that is lost. A more valuable kind of training is "just-in-time," or more in-depth training, conducted by a team facilitator as the team does its work. In this way, the information/application cycles ground new information and skills in experience. Using real data and work situations for immediate application is very valuable because it helps participants view their work and ask questions about work processes on behalf of the customers they serve.

Select the Appropriate Trainers Another consideration is selecting the appropriate trainers to deliver the material. Having managers do the training communicates the expectation that the training content will be integrated into the work. The managers and employees can immediately begin discussing together how they will use the information and tools in the real work setting.

By using managers instead of professional training staff to deliver the material, the training presentation may be somewhat compromised because managers might not have all the skills needed for making a presentation. However, the symbolism and practical integration of the manager's conveying, "This is how we work here," can be very powerful.

Evaluate the Training Experience Evaluating the impact of the training on the participants' work and relationships is part of the experience. One technique, described by Frank Navran, director of training for the National Ethics Resource Center, is to have participants leave a copy of their personal action plan in a sealed, self-addressed envelope. The trainer sends the action plan to them in three to six months with a simple survey that evaluates how well the skills have been integrated. The survey asks the following questions:[4]

- Did you put into action what you said you would?
- What changes are you making with this information?
- What changes could be made in the training to improve it for future participants?

Choose the Appropriate Team Sponsors and Facilitators

Training alone does not provide a strong enough foundation for an organization building a quality structure. To succeed, organizations must develop sponsors and facilitators who can assist improvement teams in their work.

Role of the Sponsor   Sponsorship by one of the organization's senior managers is a critical consideration in the implementation of an improvement initiative. The role of sponsor at the senior leadership level provides legitimacy to the project, gives visibility and legitimacy to the quality agenda, and keeps the specific project connected to the strategy of the organization.

The sponsor must also ensure the success of the implementation, pay attention to the process, and verify that improvement is occurring. By consistently asking the right questions, the sponsor outlines the expectations and accountabilities that ensure that change is taking place. A sponsor must ask the following questions:

- What are you changing?
- How did you come to the decisions that you've made?
- Can you talk me through the process?
- How are you using the tools?
- What is the time frame for action?

The sponsor scans the social environment to identify the resistors, saboteurs, and challengers, as well as the champions and cheerleaders of the process. Formulating strategies to specifically address detracting or negative behaviors and interactions in the improvement process is also a responsibility of the sponsor. In addition, sponsors are responsible for nurturing the energy of the team and attracting others to the team's work and contributions. Creating attractors is part of building a culture of quality. When new teams are initiated, it is important to expand the interest and energy of the team by inviting others to experience the enthusiasm of the process.

Peter Senge, among others, has advanced thinking on the topic of "initiate" and "initiation."[5] An interesting question to consider is when one "initiates," or starts, a project or improvement process, how does one invite others in the organization into the process as cocreators or participants through a process of initiation? How do you create a process or environment that attracts people to the quality agenda? The best answers to these questions are direct involvement, personal energy, enthusiasm, and active engagement of others by telling stories about the process and its results.

Ensuring that the people in the organization believe that change and improvement are necessary and possible is key to the sponsor role. Stories from other organizations that have been where you are and that have succeeded in making improvements are compelling and tangible evidence that change is possible.

Role of the Facilitator   There is strong evidence that improvement teams work more efficiently and effectively when they have guidance that supports the team's performance. The facilitator is a process expert who ensures that the team's charter has appropriate scope and definition, that the problem is precisely stated, and that the selected tools and measurements match the problem and the process. Preparing the necessary data for the team, in an understandable format consistently over time, is an essential role. In this way, the team receives the reinforcing feedback they need to advance their work.

The investments of time and intellectual capital necessary for a team process are significant. The organization develops stories based on the success or lack of success of teams, with success judged by their ability to produce results efficiently. Collectively, these stories build the organization's culture, which is reinforced or weakened by each team participant's perceptions of his or her experiences in the organization. All participants must believe that they have had the opportunity to participate and directly influence the results.

The following pitfalls in implementation undermine the quality journey:

- Taking too long; no urgency means no commitment
- Not involving the affected stakeholders
- Setting up a stand-alone program that is not integrated into organizational strategy
- Management's failing to model and to encourage others to model the quality principles

- Management's failing to connect measurements and rewards with expected behavior and results.

Sponsors and facilitators are responsible for eliminating these pitfalls.

APPLYING WHAT HAS BEEN LEARNED

Preparing people for their responsibilities in quality through training and development opportunities is only part of the work necessary to build a strong infrastructure. An organization also needs to create the processes, structures, and practices that enable people to effectively apply their knowledge and skills toward improvement efforts. This part of infrastructure ensures that learning is transferred and that processes make it easy to do good work and reward people for it.

Processes for Improvement

By constructing key self-assessment and measurement processes into the organization, leaders can ensure the ability to gauge their strengths, identify opportunities for improvement, and determine whether improvement is occurring.

Self-Assessment   Self-assessment is the first step for a quality planning process. Quality organizations submit themselves to regular, rigorous examination of their internal environment and the processes used so that they can understand and accomplish work. Self-assessment methods are used to determine the performance of a quality system—either your own or the system of a supplier or potential partner. Assessment can be done around a specific product or care site, or it can focus on the entire organization. It is the starting point for quality improvement planning because it does the following:

- Identifies opportunities
- Documents evidence of quality system implementation
- Measures effectiveness in meeting quality goals
- Measures the level of integration of the quality improvement

The definition of a self-assessment or quality assessment is a systematic and independent examination to determine whether quality activities and related results comply with established plans, whether these plans are implemented effectively, and whether they are suitable to achieve the stated objectives. An assessment compares an organization's performance to a standard, such as the Joint Commission on Accreditation of Healthcare Organizations or the National Commission on Quality Assurance, or recognized criteria, such as the Malcolm Baldrige Health Care Criteria for Performance Excellence. The aim of an assessment could include the following goals:[6]

- Obtaining factual input for a management decision
- Knowing whether the organization is at risk
- Seeing how the quality system is operating and identifying opportunity
- Assessing development and training needs
- Assessing the status and capability of equipment
- Engaging involved staff in a learning experience

A self-assessment is a rigorous and structured process that requires planning, resources, the organization's commitment to act on reported findings, and cycles of reassessment and evaluation. There are specific tools and methods for each element in the process. The results of self-assessments can be compiled to make effective quality committee and board reports.

Many organizations use the Malcolm Baldrige National Quality Award criteria for self-assessment. The Baldrige criteria, which were first adapted for health care organizations in 1995 as a pilot, provide a comprehensive mechanism for assessing and promoting performance. The criteria will be published in 1998.

Through shared learning, self-assessment provides a foundation based on the criteria's underlying values, major categories, and detailed items. The resulting assessment of current practices and performance across an organization provides a basis for identifying strengths and areas for improvement. Often, self-assessment is a prelude to strategic planning.

Measurement System Another essential component of the infrastructure for quality is the measurement system. Measures inform the organization's employees about the organization's performance; that is, whether improvement is occurring. They enable the organization's employees to learn and predict and therefore to be wise about the actions they take.

Put simply, quality measures become the gauges by which decision makers in health care organizations determine whether the organization is advancing toward the desired results. Measures also permit the observer to gauge the rate of change improvements. A balanced approach to measurement enables managers and employees to see the relationships and totality of the company operations. Typically, measures center on several perspectives: clinical quality, customer experience, core processes, innovation and learning, and economic performance. By displaying these perspectives together visually, the observer can see the interrelationships within the total company. This visual display is like the control panel in the cockpit of an airplane. It allows the observer to see a set of complex information at a glance.[7] What is measured sets the focus and gets the attention of the company. As Kaplan and Norton stated, "What is measured is what you get."[8]

If the right measures are being used, they can help managers and employees link their actions with the strategy and goals of the organization.[9] Measures provide feedback to the employees and providers at the front line for purposes of improving care and service to customers.

Purchasers and consumers of health care require that health care quality and outcomes do not suffer as a result of cost reductions.[10] Comparative data are being requested so that consumers can make informed decisions about health care choices. Regulatory and accrediting bodies have incorporated requirements that direct health care organizations to identify their quality assurance and improvement efforts and their results.[11, 12] A strategic approach to a measurement infrastructure is essential for the survival of health care organizations.

Many measurement systems fail because they contain too many detailed operational measures. Interest wanes when measures are not linked to critical business strategies. The measures must answer some critical questions: Are business strategies defined and being advanced? Is care improving? Is health improving? How do customers and stakeholders, including physicians and employees, perceive how the organization is doing? What is our rate of change? In building most measurement systems in health care, data about the organization's economic or financial performance are available. Other areas of critical information—customer feedback, physician and employee perspective, clinical quality and health improvement—are typically not as well developed and require significant effort to build.

When a health care organization develops a new measurement system, its leaders should remember that the initial goal is to stimulate new conversations and learnings about the organization's "product" and the effects of the product for the consumer. Their ultimate goal will be reaching best-in-class performance. Displays of the organization's quality measures should always include targets and clearly outlined limits, using simple, real formats. Furthermore, it is important to report quality data on a regular, anticipated schedule so that the recipients become accustomed to its arrival.

With the information provided by the measures, leaders can help executives and board members formulate questions: *Where are we? What is best-in-class? What are we doing to improve?* Together, they can use these measurements to establish clear accountabilities for improvements that underscore the measures' relevance to the organization's strategy. The inclusion of clinical measures in the measurement system is a reflection and constant reminder of the organization's real purpose—providing clinical care and health improvement.[13]

Structures to Support Information Sharing

Through the creation of structures within the organization, leaders can begin to share the knowledge and skills they have acquired, capture what has been learned by individuals throughout the organization, and bring together those responsible for carrying the information forward. A variety of structures is available, including the following:

- *Dissemination structures:* Structures for information transfer and learning are essential to quality and must be intentionally built. Dissemination strategies need to be based on the needs and learning styles of targeted audiences. Written materials, conferences, formal educational sessions and products, academic-detailing, and informational dialogues are all effective strategies. In health care, the providers are the key audience and often the most difficult to access effectively. The strategies need to be innovative, varied, and driven by what works for the provider groups. This means learning their perspective and preferences when planning dissemination strategies and recognizing that a single strategy will not be successful. This is an area in which physician champions are most helpful. Clinical colleagues communicating about what is new, helpful, and meaningful to each other is far superior to formalized organizational methods.
- *The quality initiatives directory:* The quality initiatives directory provides a data bank of key quality improvement initiatives across an organization. Each directory description should include the topic, the problem or opportunity, the methods used, results, lessons learned, and a contact person.

The directory can be used in a variety of circumstances to inform others about what has been done and to allow rapid replication and reduced cycle times. This can be especially helpful for teams that may be taking on the same or similar challenges.

- *The quality council:* The quality council can be convened with individuals from across the organization, forming a collaborative group that is focused on quality for the organization. Council members continually look outside the organization to identify best practices and innovations. The quality council also recommends the areas in which quality improvement can be used to a strategic advantage and advises on infrastructure innovations that will develop the capacity of the organization. Council members assess the progress toward reaching quality goals and gauge the progress of quality integration in the company. The council is typically chaired by the company's senior executive or the executive who leads the quality integration. The council should be solidly placed in the organization's decision-making structure, reporting to the senior leadership team responsible for operating the company. This council analyzes measurement data, looking for improvements that can be implemented across the company; sets priorities for improvement; imports new ideas and technologies; and ensures that quality is extended across the company.
- *Quality network:* A quality network is another helpful structure. Composed of quality professionals with the technical skills and implementation responsibilities to work with managers and workers at the front line, the quality network uses task forces and teams to work on specific issues.

User groups that advise and serve as resources to the rest of the organization are helpful to advance understanding on various topics. Common user groups focus on customer satisfaction measurements and key performance measurements. These groups are developmental in nature and serve to expand knowledge and skills in the topic across the organization. They become expert consumers of measurement reports and information and help interpret survey and other measurement results and their implications to colleagues.

Practices That Support Change

So that these organizational changes can truly become part of the structure of the organization, there must be policies, practices, and behaviors that support their existence and encourage their growth. Sustained organizational change is possible when the system of rewards and incentives aligns with the vision and mission. This alignment is especially visible and critical when it comes to telling—and dealing openly with—certain truths about the way things are.

Human resource policies and practices can support or undermine a quality culture. Job expectations, performance reviews, incentives, management practices, and labor management practices can support or undermine employee participation in quality. Policies and practices for working with suppliers, vendors, and partnerships also communicate the organization's commitment to quality. One example, performance reviews, is used to illustrate how these practices can "hardwire" a quality infrastructure.

Performance Reviews Policies and practices can create incentives for quality, thus advancing its progress. Performance reviews are an example. Incorporating the requirement to understand customer needs in each job description and evaluating whether employees have helped meet those needs underscore the expectation that quality principles are lived in the way work is accomplished.

Telling the truth about performance is an important element of an organization's infrastructure. Being explicit about where the organization is going and the competencies that are required gives people the information they need to see how they fit and can contribute. This means paying precise attention to the performance of people through a credible, competency-based system and giving accurate, direct feedback. It also means taking action based on the feedback, providing opportunity for development, and evaluating whether there is a "fit" between the organization and the person.[14]

Charlotte Roberts, a consultant and author, suggests the following performance review questions that a manager in an organization committed to quality and learning could use:[15]

- What do you want to accomplish during the next few years?
- What assets do you need to help accomplish this?
- What liabilities stand in your way?
- What do you need from the company to help?
- What do I do, as a manager, that gets in your way?
- What is your pattern of failure? What danger signals should I look for ahead of time, so that I know to come talk to you and help you?

The answers to these questions provide valuable information about the relationship between the employee and the manager and offer insights about the organization as a whole.

Another useful tool for evaluating a person's performance is the 360-degree performance review. This review uses the individual perspectives of an employee's leader/boss, peers, customers, and staff to create a full view of an employee's performance.

Loyalty to the Truth The policies and practices that shape the culture of the company can either support an environment that is loyal to the truth about current performance or create an environment that betrays the truth in an attempt to look better. The latter is a dangerous environment for quality. As part of the policy and practice infrastructure, Roberts has the following suggestions for organizations to follow:[16]

- Look for systemic blocks that prevent people from speaking. These can be informal punishments such as subtle put-downs and sarcasm to more formal treatment like unnecessary work tasks or sanctions.
- Provide context and training for the truth. This may be part of an ethics program or a specifically focused activity.
- When you don't speak the truth, be loyal to the spirit. This is sometimes the situation in human resources work, when confidential information cannot be divulged. A general statement, such as, "I cannot give you the specifics, but Joe and I have talked, and we feel he is not ready for this assignment yet, but I am committed to his development." This leaves little room for speculation, and the manager demonstrated candor and respect.
- Set up an amnesty policy. In setting up a quality program, people need to know there is no punishment for telling the truth. The policy should institutionalize the concept that there is no individual blame for system-related issues. In this way, data will be openly shared and reported. This works two ways. When senior executives make an error, with no intent to do wrong and they tell the truth about it, they should also be given amnesty by their board, peers, and employees.

One illustration of this is the story of the "O" ring in the U.S. Spaceship Challenger, which has become a lasting reminder that all parts of an organization must work together and invite truthful and honest communication. In the Challenger example, engineers knew of the vulnerability of the "O" ring and conditions under which it would fail, but this information never made it to the decision makers who were responsible for the launch decision. The Challenger was launched, the conditions presented themselves, and the ring failed.

Another example comes from Winston Churchill. When he discovered that Singapore was vulnerable to invasion during World War II, Churchill said, "I ought to have known. My advisors ought to have known, and I ought to have been told and ought to have asked."[17] The complexity described is enormous, but he was right—he should have known, others should have known, they should have said what they knew, and Churchill should have inquired. In an organization that is faithful to the truth and that honors those who speak it, there is an environment of respect and concern for safety, not self-protection.

These distressing examples underscore the potential tragedy in missed opportunity and error if organizational policies, procedures, and practices do not address people in organizations as individuals who are interdependent, who must act collectively, and who must communicate candidly about what they know. It is unthinkable not to do so.

CONCLUSION

This chapter outlined some key elements that should be in place to support an organization in realizing its commitment to quality. Understanding health care organization as a system and managing the system for improvement requires the know-how and skills to do it. A case study in chapter 10 illustrates how many of these infrastructure elements are applied.

References

1. Waggoner, D., et al., *Building Blocks for Quality Education and Development*, developed under a grant by Robert Wood Johnson Foundation and Pew Charitable Trust, "Strengthening Hospital Nursing—A Plan to Improve Patient Care" at Abbott Northwestern Hospital, Minneapolis, Minn., 1994.

2. Senge, P., *The Fifth Discipline* (New York: Doubleday, 1990) and Bretton Woods Conference Dialogue: Creating Learning Organizations (Summer, 1994).

3. Senge, P., et al., *The Fifth Discipline Fieldbook—Strategies for Building a Learning Organization* (New York: Doubleday, 1994).

4. Navran, F., Director of training for the National Ethics Resource Center, Washington D. C., 1997.

5. Senge, et al., 1994.

6. Waggoner, D., et al., *The Allina Tool Kit* (Allina Health System, Minnetonka, Minn., 1996).

7. Kaplan, R. S., and D. P. Norton, "The Balanced Scorecard—Measures That Drive Performance," *Harvard Business Review* 70, no. 1 (Jan.-Feb., 1992): 71–9.

8. Kaplan, R. S., and D. P. Norton, "Using the Balanced Scorecard as a Strategic Management System," *Harvard Business Review* (Jan.-Feb., 1996).

9. Kaplan and Norton, 1996.

10. Genovich-Richards, J, "The Customer: Perspectives and Expectations of Quality," In Meisenheimered, C. G., *Improving Quality: A Guide to Effective Programs* (Gaithersburg, Md.: Aspen Publishers, 1997): 133–46.

11. Joint Commission on Accreditation of Healthcare Organizations, *Manual for Hospitals* (Chicago: The Joint Commission, 1992).

12. National Committee on Quality Assurance, *Standards for the Accreditation of Managed Care Organizations,* 3rd edition (Washington, D. C.: National Committee on Quality Assurance, 1996).

13. Conversations with Paul Batalden, MD, Professor of Pediatrics, Community and Family Medicine, Dartmouth-Hitchcock Medical Center, Hanover, N.H.

14. McLagan, P., and P. Krembs, *On-the-Level-Performance Communication That Works* (St. Paul, Minn.: McLagan International, 1988).

15. Senge, et al., (1994): 220.

16. Senge, et al., (1994): 213.

17. Weick, K. E., South Canyon Revisited: Lessons from High Reliability Organizations, Wildfire, December, 1955.

Suggested Readings

Allinson, R. E., *Global Disasters* (New York: Prentice Hall, 1993): 11.

Barrentine, P., *When the Canary Stops Singing* (San Francisco: Berrett-Koehler, 1993).

Creech, B., *The Five Pillars of TQM: How to Make Total Quality Management Work for You* (New York: Truman Talley Books, 1994).

Cusimano, J. M., "Managers as Facilitators," *Training Development* 50, no. 9 (Sept., 1996): 31–3.

Davenport, T. H., *Process Innovation: Reengineering Work through Information Technology* (Boston: Harvard Business School Press, 1993).

Donovan, M., "The First Step to Self-Direction Is Not Empowerment," *The Journal for Quality and Participation* 19, no. 3 (June, 1996): 64.

Graham, M. A., and M. J. LeBaron, *The Horizontal Revolution— Reengineering Your Organization through Teams* (San Francisco: Jossey-Bass, 1994).

Green, F. B., E. Hatch, and C. Beazley, "The Road to Quality Performance Teamwork: Assessing a Firm's Progress," American Production and Inventory Control Society Conference Proceedings, 1992.

Green, F. B., "Organizational Assessment for Quality Performance Teamwork," *Self-Managed Work Teams Newsletter* 2, no. 1 (Jan., 1992): 24.

Hammer, M., and J. Champy, *Reengineering the Corporation* (New York: HarperCollins, 1993).

Hammer, M., *Beyond Reengineering* (New York: HarperCollins, 1996).

Kaluzny, A. D., C. P. McLaughlin, and D. C. Kibbe, *Continuous Quality Improvement in the Clinical Setting: Enhancing Adoption Quality Management in Health Care*, vol. 1 (Rockville, Md.: Aspen Publishers, 1992): 37–44.

Kiefer, L., "Building a Team," *Nonprofit World* 15, no. 4 (Jul.-Aug., 1997): 39–41.

Lawler, E. E., S. A. Mohrman, and G. E. Ledord, *Employee Involvement and Total Quality Management Practices and Results in Fortune 1000 Companies* (San Francisco: Jossey-Bass, 1992).

"Organizing for Quality—Implementation Guide," *FACCT, The Foundation for Accountability,* 1997.

Palmer, P. J., *The Courage to Teach* (San Francisco: Jossey-Bass, 1998.

Senge, P., et al., *The Fifth Discipline Fieldbook* (New York: Bantam Doubleday, 1994): 446.

Shronk, J. H., *Team-Based Organizations: Developing a Successful Team Environment* (Homewood, Ill.: Business One, 1992).

Simons, R., *Levers of Control* (Boston: Harvard Business School Press, 1995).

Wellins, R. S., W. C. Byham, and G. R. Dixon, *Inside Teams—How 20 World-Class Organizations Are Winning through Teams* (San Francisco: Jossey-Bass, 1994).

Vitale, K. F., "Teams—the Essence of Quality," *Nonprofit World* 13(3) (May-June, 1995): 47–50.

6

Making Change Happen

It takes courage to confront reality and act on it. Leaders who pay attention to their company's ongoing performance measures and seek out the stories and experiences behind those measures are those with the edge to see how things really are within their organizations. The actual picture of performance is often obscured in rhetoric. Knowing what is important to the organization, demanding rigorous measures of what is important, and knowing the organization's performance against the best-of-class performers provide leaders with the evidence to make tough decisions and focus the organization toward what needs to be done for a stronger future. Understanding the customers and anticipating their needs, as well as looking inside at the organization's performance, allow leaders to see the gap and generate the kind of creative tension that can focus energy and drive action.[1] The ability to use this energy to take direct action, to make it clear to people "what mountain they are to climb," is what Jack Welch, CEO of General Electric, identified as "the edge."[2] The edge requires seeing and telling the truth, which includes admitting failure.

This chapter discusses the benefits of accomplishing change quickly and identifies the conditions that must exist for change to occur. It then uses a case study at Allina Health System to illustrate how a care improvement model might be designed, communicated, and implemented. Finally, organizational culture as the context for taking action to improve quality is discussed.

BENEFITS OF MAKING CHANGE HAPPEN QUICKLY

Urgency and impatience are necessary to achieve "the edge" to create changes in improvement and realize results rapidly. As Dr.

111

Robert Panzer, Chief Quality Officer and Associate Medical Director for the University of Rochester Medical Center and Strong Memorial Hospital said, "Accelerated improvement is better than slow improvement. It gets things done before the solution changes and while the team still has energy to implement its ideas."[3]

This opinion is expressed across the health care industry. There is increasing concern about and frustration around the protracted cycle times for change that are inherent in the traditional, research-based change methodology that seems to have been applied to every circumstance. Improvement processes that take too long are at the greatest risk for failure.[4] Failure results in waste, unrealized benefits, frustrated people, and unmet customer need.

Using methods to accelerate or increase the speed at which quality improvement occurs means getting better and faster at meeting the needs and preferences of customers. It also has the benefit of sustaining and encouraging the energy of teams who can see a clear path toward desired results, an end point, and the results of their efforts in their lifetime.

Story of Two Teams

Two improvement teams were asked to relate critical factors in their experience with a process improvement effort.[5] One team had been in place for more than 1,460 days without producing an improvement. They declared this process a slow process. In contrast, the second team worked for nine days and improved the product—a fast process. Figure 6-1 shows factors that team members said characterized each process.

The factors associated with prolonged cycle times were employee perceptions that the organization lacked commitment and support, the know-how to create change, and the resources to help. The involved employees were cynical about whether the leadership of the organization was serious about change and improvement. On the other hand, the nine-day cycle time of improvement was associated with supportive leadership and competent, confident, and empowered employees.

Lessons Learned

What can be learned from these two experiences? The first lesson is obtained by examining figure 6-1 and noting the conditions identified by the slow process team. These could be called conditions

FIGURE 6-1. Factors That Characterized the Process of a Fast Team and a Slow Team

Slow—Pace-Limiting Factors	Fast—Speed Factors
Mixed loyalties and commitment to an outcome by members: • Hidden agenda • Political process Unclear/lack of accountability for results: • Time • Authority • Ability to implement Unclear/absent commitment of resources to implement Absence of senior leadership sponsorship; unclear messages Lack of staff support Lack of focus • Definition of project scope kept changing Environment changed Definition of problem changed No team formation: • Inconsistent participation • No preparation for team members • Turnover in team members No time frame Back-tracking and rework Data needs not met Not connected to strategy	Common enemy—urgency Problem of strategic importance Shared vision for desired outcome Focus Senior management commitment Just-in-time training Clear charter Dedicated team Expert facilitation Data

Reprinted, with permission, from Allina Health System, Minnetonka, Minn., 1998.

for failure to be aware of and to avoid. Teams need to be chartered to improve areas of strategic importance. These areas must have tangible and visible senior sponsorship and leadership. Quality improvement is the science of process management. A body of knowledge and discipline of practice surround improvement and change and need to be faithfully applied. Forming a group activity to improve an area of function without the knowledge and expertise needed for effective improvement can set back quality improvement efforts. Well-intentioned people and actions, without the proper foundation, can undermine the very principles of quality improvement.

Dr. Brian Anderson, a cardiologist and frequent speaker on the topic of quality, describes "a group as people you have coffee with and a team as people you produce results with."[6] A team is prepared, focused, and results-oriented. The final lesson is that a commitment to quality is also a commitment to invest in expertise and resources, particularly information. It is also a commitment to build the infrastructure to support the work of improvement. And again, the lesson for leaders is that they must be out in front, leading.

CONDITIONS FOR EFFECTIVE TRANSITION OR CHANGE

Tichey and Cohen have catalogued five conditions that must exist for effective transitions or changes to take place. Although leaders might not personally create the conditions, they must ensure that the following conditions exist:[7]

1. A sense of urgent need that is clear and palpable to everyone in the organization
2. A mission that is inspiring and clearly worth achieving
3. Goals that stretch people's ability
4. A spirit of teamwork—a sense that "we are all in this together"
5. A realistic expectation that people can meet the goals

Successful leaders create the need for change so that the focus and energy that already exist in a successful organization are increased. For example, Alcoa CEO, Paul O'Neill, said the company will focus on safety first, when no other company in the industry was doing so. Jack Welch said that General Electric would put quality first; Bill George challenged Medtronic to levels of unsurpassed quality. Recall the focus of the aerospace industry, when President John F. Kennedy stated that the United States would have the first man on the moon. Leaders neither create inconsequential change nor do they fail to recognize or create essential change. They do not allow people to hold onto identities, behavior, or practices at the expense of failing to meet the emerging needs of customers and to reach the vision of the company. Small- or large-scale change, intelligently focused, is a recurring theme in the practice of quality leaders.

REJECTION OF THE STATUS QUO

Letting go of the past is a particular interest in health care quality. Failure to find new ways in merged organizations, joint ventures, and complex relationships is unacceptable. Waste is generated when employees go through motions without producing a product that meets the needs of customers. Getting on with change, letting go of the past, and focusing on the patient and health plan member are collective obligations. Health care is an industry with deep roots, with practices that have been transferred from generation to generation largely through apprenticeships. Evidence-based practice and attention to routine, not blind repetition, are still emerging approaches to the care process.

The foundation of the health care organization, the provider-patient relationship, is changing. Making the commitment to quality as a business strategy also means making the commitment to changing how care is delivered.

COMPONENTS OF SUCCESSFUL CHANGE EFFORTS

The following list of 10 components of successful, rapid change efforts was published in *The Quality Letter.*[8]

1. A desire or mandate to finish the project quickly
2. A clear aim
3. A way to measure performance
4. Access to exciting research
5. Good data collection on site, analysis, and project management
6. Support from leadership
7. A willingness to make incremental changes
8. The ability to do quick, small-scale tests
9. Impatience
10. These, plus the need for team skill development and effective facilitation, are criteria to consider when engaging a team with the task of improving a process.

The following case study of clinical change is authored by Dr. Robert Jeddeloh, Associate Medical Director of Public Programs and Director of Care System Innovation at Allina Health Systems (AHS).[9] The case study demonstrates the focus, design, use of infrastructure, and role of leadership in improving a care process. It illustrates the 10 components of successful, rapid change. In this case study, the breakthrough series methodology was selected to achieve successful rapid change.

DESIGN AND SYSTEMATIC APPROACH FOR IMPROVEMENT: A CASE STUDY

This case study illustrates that improvement is not just a matter of will, but also a matter of skill to design, communicate, and select tools and processes that enable change to improve care. AHS became involved in the development and support of a health clinic in an urban elementary school. The school nurse relayed a series of stories compelling enough to prompt an examination of potential improvements in the way care was delivered in this school setting. Asthma was one clinical condition that adversely affected students. The school nurse reported that students often sought care in the emergency departments of nearby hospitals and that 20 percent of the school's students missed school because of poorly controlled asthma.

Focus Priorities

Claims data for health plan members attending the elementary school were examined to gain additional information about care patterns. One fourth grader's claims history confirmed the impact of asthma: four emergency department visits, one resulting in hospital admission, for one six-month period. During that same period, no claims were made for clinical visits and no steroid anti-inflammatory inhalers were prescribed. However, multiple β-agonist inhalers had been prescribed. The claims history showed a pattern of acute exacerbations and emergency care and the absence of any ongoing primary care relationship. This single claims history highlighted that, although the optimal treatment of asthma is well described and guidelines and new medications have been shown to improve the outcomes and reduce the cost of asthma care, this child was not receiving the optimal recommended care.[10]

The impact of asthma on the members and patients of AHS led to the identification of pediatric asthma as one of Allina's clinical priorities. Asthma met the following three essential components for selection:

1. High impact on quality and cost
2. Practice patterns that can be changed
3. Availability of measurable results

Define the Work

A best-of-practice panel convened to examine the evidence-based information related to asthma care. A team of allergists, pulmonologists, and primary care practitioners followed a comprehensive process to identify position papers, nationally recognized guidelines and policy statements, locally available guidelines, and bibliographies of recognized and acknowledged contributors to the care and management of asthma. This extensive review process, coordinated by a member of the quality team, defined the key requirements of "ideal" asthma care and pointed out gaps in the current patterns of care. The group confirmed that guidelines and standards of care for inpatient, emergency department, outpatient, specialist, and primary care practices were available and yet were not uniformly applied.

Mobilize Action-Takers

Once the evidence was reviewed and an optimal pattern of care identified, a multidisciplinary expert panel of practitioners, called the Pediatric Asthma Clinical Action Group (CAG), convened. Chaired by an allergist and a pediatric pulmonologist, the goal of CAG was to reduce the burden of asthma on the children and families of Minnesota. The group members included those practitioners recognized as experts by their peers and those who cared for a large number of health plan members with asthma. These practitioners came from multiple health systems in the area. The group's challenge was twofold: to clarify the key clinical outcomes and the objectives needed to accomplish the best practices already identified and to examine the data for information that would enable practitioners at the point of care and the CAG members to measure progress and their success. Data reviewed included economic impact, noneconomic impact such as missed days from school, prescribing patterns of physicians, member "compliance" to diagnostic and treatment regimens, and frequency and site of care information.

Community-oriented from the outset, the group set out to examine strategic problems and opportunities and to propose key actions and recommendations to ensure optimal outcomes of care. The group examined areas where variation in care was thought to occur and where the cost of poor quality was of most concern. They accepted the challenge of examining why the new and accepted knowledge of asthma care had not spread to all the people who could benefit and why there was no effective, integrated community approach to the delivery of asthma care. A school nurse, a public health nurse, and asthma educators routinely challenged the group to focus on an integrated, community-based approach to the care of asthma. Questions such as the following continually challenged the group's thinking:

- "Why can't a student get the same medications in school as at home?"
- "Why can't education materials in the doctor's office be the same as those in the hospital or the school?"

These practitioners reminded the group that each child with asthma lives in a community of family, friends, schools, and other social support systems that affect that child's ability to cope with asthma. They challenged the CAG to move outside of the traditional medical and public health models to look at a community model of integrated asthma care.

Set Goals and Targets

The CAG articulated four major goals that would address the gaps in asthma care they had identified. They continue to work to ensure dissemination and to develop and test action plans and pilots that focus on the most effective way to reach the following goals.

1. Provide consistent, well-timed, and ongoing education for patients and their families, health care providers, health system administrators, managers, and executives.
2. Create and implement a chronic disease management model for asthma that incorporates the strengths of existing models and that includes a registry of people with asthma and linkages to a care management system that ensures ongoing care and evaluation.
3. Improve the identification and diagnosis of asthma, and develop standardized language to describe asthma and asthma severity.
4. Partner with schools, school districts, and area health plans to develop and coordinate a comprehensive in-school asthma care program.

The accomplishment of each of these goals required the engagement of practitioners from throughout the community, not just those affiliated with AHS. Building and maintaining the necessary working relationships were identified as necessary parts of any action plan. The CAG work included the process of identifying the key tasks and actions in the next steps. Work teams were formed, and targeted pilot programs were designed.

Implement Recommendations

The implementation of the CAG recommendations was built on the principles and practice of continuous quality improvement. Dr. Donald Berwick, a champion of continuous quality improvement (through the Institute for Healthcare Improvement Breakthrough Series "Improving Asthma Care in Children and Adults") outlines a deceptively simple model for producing system change through rapid improvement cycles. See figure 6-2.

FIGURE 6-2. The Model for Improvement

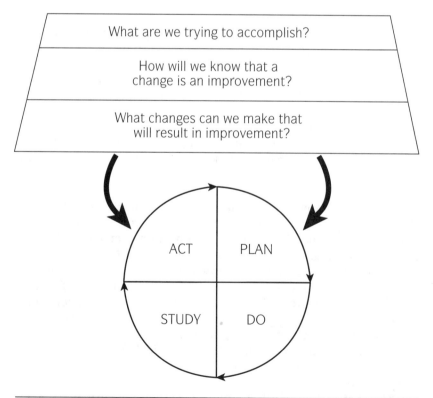

Reprinted, with permission, from G. J. Langley, K. M. Nolan, T. W. Nolan, C. Norman, and L. P. Provost, *The Improvement Guide: A Practical Approach to Enhancing Organizational Performance* (San Francisco: Jossey-Bass, 1996).

FIGURE 6-3.   Repeated Use of the Cycle

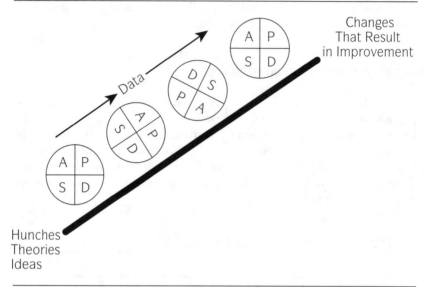

Reprinted, with permission, from G. J. Langley, K. M. Nolan, T. W. Nolan, C. Norman, L. P. Provost, *The Improvement Guide: A Practical Approach to Enhancing Organizational Performance* (San Francisco: Jossey-Bass, 1996).

The following three questions drive the process:[11]

1. What are we trying to accomplish?
2. How will we know that a change is an improvement?
3. What changes can we make that will result in an improvement?

A series of progressive cycles of experimentation based on the Plan, Do, Study, Act cycle of process improvement help answer the questions. Students of continuous quality improvement will recognize the ongoing, repetitive nature of this cycle to drive from hunches, theories, and good ideas to changes that result in real improvement in the processes of care. Data and measurement form the foundation for the cycles; the ongoing collection and reflection on information informs and drives the action elements of the cycle. A series of cycles, as illustrated in figure 6-3, builds a ramp to change.[12] At each meeting, a work team can ask practical questions that form the basis for the model:

- What is the smallest number (patients, health plan members, encounters, surveys, and so on) that will test an idea?

- What can a small group of people or one individual accomplish by next Tuesday?

In this framework, the process of improvement becomes the task and the responsibility of each individual and each work team. Each turn of the cycle produces a measurable outcome.

Select Appropriate Measures

Measurement and reflection on the information collected forms the foundation of improvement. The CAG wrestled with what information it would need to judge the success of any action related to the individual goals. By a process of discussion and elimination, the group grappled with the information systems currently available and what information elements they believed would most directly affect those people involved in asthma care. The following indicators were selected:

1. Asthma inpatient admission rate
2. Rate of children with asthma who had one, two, three, or more emergency department admissions
3. Rate of children with asthma who had two or more emergency department visits and who had a prescription for steroid inhalers or mast cell stabilizers after their second visit
4. Rate of children with asthma who are compliant with care recommendations
5. Cost per member, per month for children with severe (two or more emergency department visits) and less severe (fewer than two emergency department visits) asthma
6. Rate of parents of children with asthma who reported the following via study survey:
   - Having and using a written asthma plan
   - Being satisfied with overall care
   - Having a peak flow meter for their child

Indicators 1, 2, 3, and 5 could be measured by using the existing data systems in Allina facilities. Indicators 4 and 6 required the use of a stratified sampling methodology by survey. The use of surveys could be coordinated and integrated into those already used at the point of care. The combination of objective utilization data and the survey data would, the group believed, provide a way to watch improvement over time as action items were tested and implemented.

Sharing the information with clinicians could provide an ongoing measure of practice change.

Use Measurement to Drive Change

The team used the principles of data use measurement articulated by Thomas Nolan, PhD (IHI Breakthrough Series). The overriding principle is that measurements are useful to speed things up, not to slow them down. The following principles were followed:[13]

- Seek usefulness, not perfection. Measurement is not the goal, improvement is. A work team needs just enough measurement to know whether changes are leading to improvement in order to move forward to the next step.
- Don't wait for the information system. Useful information already exists or is relatively simple to get. Don't wait for the financial figures to come out two months or more from now, or for surveys to come back in two weeks.
- Use sampling, a simple and powerful way to help understand how a system is working. Instead of measuring all of something, measure a sample—every 10th patient, or the next 10 patients, or the next 30 bills.
- Use qualitative and quantitative data. Ask the caregivers: "What are the top three or four reasons for asthma education not working?" "Why do you think peak flow meters aren't being used in the emergency department?" These qualitative judgments can be certified and data can be collected during tests of change.

With these principles for the use of measurement, rapid cycle change can move forward, supported by data and information, rather than be impeded and bogged down by countless reasons for "not having data."

Implement the Model for Changing the Process

A model of integrated asthma care, developed through action plans and implementations steps, is evolving on the following five levels, which Weiss describes as levels of competence and capacity.[14]

1. Patient-clinician competence
2. Multidisciplinary clinical competence

3. Multidomain (clinical and nonclinical) capacity
4. System services integration
5. Disease-state (population) management capacity

Each level requires the participation of multiple practitioners dedicated to working toward improved asthma care. Work at each level requires building capacity for action and change. Examples of action items proposed by the CAG and work already in progress help illustrate each level, the interrelatedness and complexity of the process, and the ability to affect care.

Level 1: Patient-Clinician Competence Patient-clinician competence speaks to Goal 1 of the CAG: "To provide consistent and well-timed education to providers, patients, and families." Action to accomplish this goal needs to plan, carry out, and measure the effectiveness of efforts to build on the knowledge, attitudes, and beliefs of patients and their families and clinical providers.

The CAG identified that education should be a priority of initial efforts. A subgroup searched for and examined those education efforts and materials that were currently available. The group's intent will be to target specific materials to the specific needs of patients and their families at various stages of managing asthma.

One project already under way is the Inner City Asthma Camp Program, the Family Asthma Experience, sponsored by the American Lung Association of Hennepin County, the National Consortium of Asthma Camps, and Allina. The goal of the program is to involve community residents and families in a creative, innovative, and interactive format to increase knowledge and management of asthma.

Pilot projects proposed by the subset of the CAG, asthma educators, and community-based practitioners target specific clinic practices or community settings as did the "Family Asthma Experience," so that they can build and measure the effectiveness of tools to increase self-knowledge about asthma care.

Level 2: Multidisciplinary Clinical Competence Multidisciplinary clinical competence builds on the relationship between the clinical provider and patients and their families to involve other providers such as emergency department caregivers, specialist care staff, respiratory care staff, and health educators in the clinical setting. Essential to this work are effective hand-off mechanisms from one level of care to another.

An action team that grew out of the "Breakthrough Series on Asthma Care" focuses on asthma care in the emergency department. Work team members from throughout the community are using the rapid-cycle improvement model to see what they can accomplish in a community-wide setting. The group accepted the challenge and reported at the National Congress for Asthma Care sponsored by the Institute for Health Care Improvement. Initial survey work examined care relative to two variables: use of a peak flow meter and the prescription of anti-inflammatory medications. Chart review of a limited sample (20) from several emergency departments indicated that there was room for improvement. The group was also able to report on the complexity of scheduling, team dynamics, and organization-related frustrations that result from working across multiple health care systems. The team renewed its pledge to move forward with the work, broaden the scope of measurement by survey to confirm the initial results, and begin the recruitment of emergency department staffs to build their own CAGs.

Level 3: Community Capacity   The community (clinical and nonclinical) capacity builds on levels 1 and 2 to involve the components of an entire health system and community support such as schools. Working toward the CAG goals of (1) a chronic disease management model for asthma and (2) partnering with schools, school districts, and area health plans occurs at the third level.

Based on the principles of chronic disease management, a model for disease management for asthma requires resources such as care management and integration with services at clinics and home care agencies. The results from a pilot were used to measure the success of a care management process on improving asthma self-knowledge and care. The pilot developed, tested, and implemented a selection tool that used functional status to identify members with moderate and severe asthma. Care management staff targeted specific strategies to the needs that members identified. Follow-up at two weeks and three months demonstrated improved self-knowledge of asthma and a decrease in the cost of acute care in emergency departments and hospitals. The number of project members was expanded, and a cost-benefit analysis of the model was developed.

Another work team from the CAG examined the policies and procedures for asthma care that existed in schools. Partnerships will be developed with school district staffs who are interested in improving asthma care, and sites will be recruited to participate in local CAG teams. One site already up and running is the health clinic currently in place at the urban elementary school referenced in this case study.

Level 4: System Services Integration   The integration of system services means more coordination, communication, and dissemination of information. Information on pilots and strategies will help build and spread the process improvement to a broader audience.

Successes and failures provide critical knowledge. Dissemination of information through the educational resources of the company and links to other health systems will help spread successful implementations of this model and speed replication.

Level 5: Disease-State Management Capacity   The ability to manage a population of patients with the same disease builds on an organization's service integration. Characterizing a population requires that they be stratified by asthma severity, with intervention strategies targeted for each. That is, programs with high efficacy and high cost are targeted to those with the most severe disease, and the least efficacious and least costly programs are targeted to a broader audience with mild disease.

With this level of management, those six to seven percent of asthma patients who presently require 45 to 55% of the asthma resources can be anticipated, identified, and offered personalized care. This level of management requires a disease registry that is accessible at the point of care; knowledge of specific targeted interventions by each clinical provider; and accepted nomenclature for severity, supported with coding methodology. With this level of population management, the goals of the CAG can be realized.

The CAG recognizes that the information system support needed to build such capacity will not be readily available in one piece. The development of an electronic medical record provides a way to start piloting and building successful components of such a system.

Assess Results

The Allina clinical care model has used the company's infrastructure and the structure of the Institute for Health Improvement as the support for an action-focused infrastructure and as a way to engage 100 clinical and community providers of asthma care in a defined process with the goal of improving the care of children with asthma. The CAG has articulated goals and objectives and is in the process of defining discrete action items to build toward an integrated model of care. Several pilot projects are already under way, and additional pilots are planned for implementation. Each builds on a quality improvement model of Plan, Do, Study, and Act to ensure thoughtful design and planning, measurement, reflection, effectiveness, and success. The challenge is to coordinate the work of the individual teams, build on pilots and tests, communicate work in progress success, and be able to build a model that affects the community and reaches the goal of improved asthma care.

CULTURAL CONTEXT FOR ACTION

When thinking about implementing and accelerating quality improvement, Mary Alice Jordan-Marsh, RN, PhD, FAAN, from the University of Southern California, Los Angeles, reminds action-takers to reflect on the content of their Anthropology 101 course work and realize that implementation takes place in the context of a culture—the values, norms, and customs of a group.[15] The start of a pain management improvement initiative in Jordan-Marsh's organization was a call-to-arms to be "cutting edge," a distinguishing feature of that organization's culture. Following a consultation about the emerging evidence for pain management, she returned to her agency and announced that, "We are all behind. No one is giving intramuscular injections for pain anymore." Although she has since clarified the consultant's exact message, her message created the energy the agency needed to learn about, improve, and reduce variance in the management of pain. The organization's cultural value of being on "the cutting edge" did not tolerate the possibility that the agency was not leading the way in this area. Jordan-Marsh tapped the energy of her culture to mobilize for action. This is what Chip Caldwell of the Juran Institute refers to as building the burning platform for change.[16] This involves creating a compelling reason for change and improvement that strikes a resonant chord with the values of the organization.

Because change takes place in the context of an organization's culture, a brief discussion of culture and health care organizations is presented here. Dr. John Kleinman, Vice President of Clinical Services, Allina Health System, has identified the following four attributes of health care organizations that are more effective at encouraging people to take action and implement change.[17]

1. *A group culture:* This culture is oriented toward interdisciplinary and team function in which people cross professional and departmental boundaries to focus on shared organizational goals, based on what the customer needs and prefers. This is a culture of mutual respect and contribution.
2. *A culture of learning:* This culture is characterized by exploration to understand better ways of working, humility to ask

for more information, and an admission of not having all the answers. The system invests in learning and creates safe places for people to think and learn together. The learning is focused on what the organization needs to be good at, in this case, improving health care and reducing the burden of illness.

3. *An information-based culture:* In this culture, data are gathered, analyzed, and used consistently for decision making. The members of this culture have an insatiable appetite for information about how they are doing, what is best or better practice, and what the benchmarks are to reach their goals. This culture is skilled at getting timely and relevant information to the front line.

4. *A risk-sharing culture:* This culture accepts risk to improve the health care and experiences of a population(s). These attributes form a helpful framework for assessing an organization's readiness.

Richard Edelson, DDS, Director of the Minneapolis Education Center and VA Employee Education System, has done considerable work around the question of culture and improvement. He consistently cautions that when considering the culture, it is essential to assess and fully appreciate the enabling factors in the work environment that support behavioral changes over time, such as feedback systems and incentives that reward and recognize improvement.[18] He is pursuing the following questions: How does an organization gain assurance that improvement is not a single, brilliant leap of improvement that is subsequently abandoned? How does an organization ensure that improvement is continuous over time?

These are questions about the infrastructure necessary for quality. The following example illustrates how a project is integrated into the fabric of the organization through its infrastructure. Implementation of Agency for Health Care Policy and Research's (AHCPR) pain guidelines was a quality improvement initiative for the home care division of the Allina Health System in Minnetonka, Minnesota. Following the initial dissemination of the AHCPR Pain Guideline Project, Dr. Edward Ratner, Home Care Medical Director, led a strategic planning process that advanced pain management as a key strategy of the home care division. Formal measurements of competence in pain assessment and management were developed and integrated into the professional staff performance expectations and evaluations. Both of these strategies wove the concepts of focus and discipline in pain management into the fabric of the home care division's operational systems.

CONCLUSION

This chapter discussed the conditions required for action to produce the desired results. Leadership that is fluent in what conditions currently are and has a vision of what they can be will provide the urgency and energy that the people in the organization need to move toward a shared vision and common goals. Committing to a disciplined process and investing in the expertise and infrastructure for improvement provide the pathway and know-how to channel energy so that the desired results can be achieved. To do less is to lose the edge necessary to achieve success. A case study was used to illustrate what a large scale and complex improvement process can look like. Speed and acceleration of change were themes throughout. Culture was introduced as the context in which action is taken. The following chapters expand on the infrastructure for improvement and the role of measurement.

References

1. Senge, P., *The Fifth Discipline* (New York: Doubleday, 1990).

2. Tichey, N., and E. Cohen, *The Leadership Engine: How Winning Companies Build Leaders at Every Level* (New York: Harper-Collins, 1997): 153.

3. O'Malley, S., "Total Quality Now! Putting QI on the Fast Track," *The Quality Letter* 9, no. 11 (Dec., 1997): 3.

4. Caldwell C., author of *Mentoring Strategic Change in Health Care* and Vice President of the Juran Institute, Rapid Acceleration, a workshop conducted for Allina Health System, Minnetonka, Minn. (Oct., 1997).

5. Allina Health System, Minnetonka, Minn., 1997.

6. Anderson, B., MD, practicing cardiologist and frequent consultant and speaker on quality, Heart Center, Mercy Hospital, Coon Rapids, Minn., for Allina Health System.

7. Tichey and Cohen, p. 153.

8. O'Malley, S., "Total Quality Now: Putting OI on the Fast Track," *The Quality Letter for Healthcare Leaders* 9, no. 11 (Dec., 1997): 2–10.

9. Jeddeloh, R., MD, Associate Medical Director of Public Programs and Director of Care System Innovation, Allina Health System, Minnetonka, Minn., 1998. Unpublished case study.

10. NHLBI Guidelines, *Annals of Internal Medicine* 126, no. 10 (May, 1997): 146–7.

11. Langley, G. J., K. M. Nolan, and T. W. Norlan, *API: The Foundation of Improvement*, abstract presented at the Institute for Health Improvement, "Linking Outcome Measurement and Clinical Quality Course" (Jan., 1998): 4.

12. Langley, Nolan, and Norlan.

13. Langley, G., et al., *The Improvement Guide: A Practical Approach to Enhancing Organizational Performance* (San Francisco, Jossey-Bass, 1996).

14. Weiss, K. B., ed. National Asthma Education and Prevention Program Task Force Report on the Cost-Effectiveness, Quality of Care, and Financing of Asthma Care. Supplement to *American Journal of Respiratory Care Medicine* 154 (3 pt 2) (Sept., 1996): 96–118.

15. Jordan-Marsh, M. A., RN, PhD, FAAN (Faculty, University of Southern California, Los Angeles), interview with author, Oct., 1997.

16. Caldwell.

17. Kleinman, J., MD (Vice President, Allina Health System, Minnetonka, Minn.), interview with author, 1997.

18. Edelson, R., DDS (Director, Minneapolis Education Center and VA Employee Education System), interview with author, 1997.

Suggested Readings

Brailer, D. J., et al., "Physician-Led Clinical Performance Improvement: A Model for Quality Management," *Journal of Clinical Outcomes Management* 4, no. 5 (1997): 33–43.

Caldwell, C., ed., *The Handbook for Managing Change in Health Care* (Milwaukee: ASQ Quality Press, 1998).

Caldwell, C., *Mentoring Strategic Change in Health Care* (Milwaukee: ASQ Quality Press, 1995).

Deming, W. E., *Out of the Crisis* (Cambridge, Mass.: Massachusetts Institute of Technology, 1986).

First National Quality of Care Forum, "Bridging the Gap Between Theory and Practice," Hospital Research and Educational Trust and the Parke-Davis Division of the Warner-Lambert Company, May 14–15, 1992, Chicago.

Gavin, D. A., *Managing Quality: The Strategic and Competitive Edge* (New York: Free Press, 1988).

Grossman, S., "Turning Technical Groups into High-Performance Teams," *Research-Technology Management* 40, no. 2 (Mar.-Apr., 1997): 9–11.

Gustafson, D., Accelerating Quality Improvement Feature, *The Quality Letter for Healthcare Leaders* 9, no. 11 (Dec., 1997):13–14.

Holpp, L., "It's All in the Planning," *Training and Development* 51, no. 4 (Apr., 1997): 44–7.

Horak, B., *Strategic Planning in Healthcare—Building a Quality-Based Plan Step-by-Step* (New York: Quality Resource, Kraus Organization, 1997).

James, B., "Implementing Practice Guidelines through CQI," *Frontiers of Health Service Management* 10, no. 1 (Fall, 1993): 3–37.

Kaluzny, A. D., C. P. McLaughlin, and D. C. Kibbe, "Continuous Quality Improvement in the Clinical Setting: Enhancing Adoption," *Quality Management in Health Care* 1, no. 1 (1992): 37–44.

Mariotti, J. L., *The Shape Shifters: Continuous Change for Competitive Advantage* (New York: Van Nostrand Reinhold, 1997).

Moen, R. D., and T. W. Nolan, "Process Improvement," *Quality Progress* 20, no. 9 (Sept., 1987): 62–8.

Moen, R. D., T. W. Nolan, and L. P. Provost, *Improving Quality through Planned Experimentation* (New York: McGraw-Hill, 1991).

Nolan, T., and D. Berwick, "Understanding Medical Systems, Physicians As Leaders in Improving Health Care," *American College of Physicians* 128 (Feb., 1998): 289–90.

Parry, C., et al., "Putting Best Practices into Practice," *The Systems Thinker* 8, no. 10 (Dec., 1997-Jan., 1998): 1–5.

Robison, J., "Integrate Quality Cost Concepts into Teams' Problem-Solving Efforts," *Quality Progress* 30, no. 3 (Mar., 1997): 25–30.

Rogers, E. M., *Diffusion of Innovations,* 4th edition (New York: The Free Press, 1995).

Shewhart, W. A., *The Economic Control of Quality of Manufactured Product.* (New York: D. Van Nostrand Company, 1931, reprinted by the American Society of Quality Control, 1980).

Shortell, S., "High-Performing Healthcare Organizations: Guidelines for Pursuit of Excellence," *Hospital and Health Services Administration* 30, no. 4 (July-Aug., 1985): 7–35.

von Bertalanffy, L., *General Systems Theory* (New York: George Braziller, 1968).

Wheeler, D. J., and D. S. Chambers, *Understanding Statistical Process Control* (Knoxville, Tenn.: Statistical Process Controls, 1992).

7

Selecting a Focus and Getting Started

Joachim Roski, PhD

Many health care organizations have begun to seriously address the elimination of waste in their administrative and client/patient service processes. Reducing telephone wait times, responding more quickly to customer complaints and resolving them speedily, and redesigning admitting or billing processes to make them more customer friendly are tactics that have been pursued, often resulting in quick improvements. However, redesigning clinical processes and care delivery has generally proven to be much more difficult and, as a result, has rarely been the initial improvement focus for health care organizations committed and ready to begin to continuously improve quality.

This chapter introduces several criteria that health care organizations need to consider when deciding which clinical areas to focus on for the greatest results. In addition, it briefly introduces methods that might assist a health care organization's senior management in reaching these kinds of decisions.

OVERCOMING RELUCTANCE TO ENGAGE IN CLINICAL CARE IMPROVEMENTS

The motivation of health care organizations to improve processes has often been economic rather than driven by a desire to enhance customers' or patients' experiences or their clinical outcomes. However, nurses and physicians are often less inspired by achieving cost efficiencies than they are by the potential of improving a patient's well-being. Thus, redesign efforts that are undertaken to remove only cost and waste from the system are less likely to foster clinician and physician enthusiasm. The reasons behind this reluctance to engage in clinical care improvements are manifold. The redesign of clinical processes and patient care must include the intense involvement of clinicians and physicians, an aspect that often proves to be difficult. Redesign of clinical processes is mostly pursued with the goal of reducing unwarranted clinical variation. This is sometimes negatively perceived by physicians as an attempt to reduce their decision-making autonomy.

Unwarranted clinical variation accounts for major waste and substandard patient care. For example, Wennberg[1] demonstrated that the likelihood of women receiving radical hysterectomies in neighboring New England counties is almost twice as high from one county to the other, even though patients had very similar sociodemographic and clinical characteristics. It has been estimated that not more than 20 percent of current medical practice is research based, with most clinical care being determined by physicians' individual experiences and opinions or community care standards.[2-4] On one hand, clinical variation might be ethically defensible when research evidence is not unequivocal or nonexistent. On the other hand, even when research evidence about the benefits or harmful consequences of particular procedures is available, these care processes are not consistently delivered. For example, even though the benefits of identifying smoking status and giving brief, firm advice to quit have been shown to be of great benefit in dramatically decreasing smoking among patients, fewer than half of smokers recall their physicians ever asking them if they are smokers or advising them to quit smoking.[5]

SELECTING CLINICAL AREAS OF FOCUS

The effort to improve clinical care quality and its outcomes can easily become an overwhelming endeavor given the hundreds of clinical conditions, dozens of associated clinical care processes, and huge outlays of financial and human resources that each targeted process potentially requires. Thus, it becomes essential to focus on just a few conditions that the organization considers important for being able to affect the quality of care. However, what criteria should be used to select areas of clinical focus and improvement are often less clear.

A mission-driven organization will want to ensure that its clinical areas of focus or "clinical product lines" are tied to its vision and mission to ensure direction and constancy of purpose. Vision and mission statements differ among various types of health care organizations. For example, a public health–oriented organization such as a health department is likely to define its mission differently than a health maintenance organization or a hospital. In addition, the vision and mission statements of hospitals might differ among similar organizations. For example, rural hospitals might emphasize different missions than metropolitan hospitals that specialize in highly evolved tertiary care.

In addition to linking clinical foci to the organization's mission, it is helpful to conduct an analysis of the external environment in which the organization operates, such as gaining an understanding of the strategies and activities of competitors, legislators, and health care consumers. Such an analysis can help guide in the selection of clinical focus areas to ensure the relevancy of the selected conditions to important stakeholders, such as legislators and customers/ patients, and to competitively position the organization.

A number of criteria should be considered when selecting an organization's clinical areas of focus. Although there are no clearly identifiable methods for weighing the relative importance of these criteria, the considerations can be grouped into four major areas of knowledge: clinical condition, improvability, customer understanding, and organizational understanding.

Clinical Condition

A range of data should be taken into account under the heading clinical condition. First, the *prevalence and incidence* of the clinical condition need to be considered. How many individuals are likely to be affected by this condition, and how many new cases can be expected during defined time intervals? Both publicly available information, such as incidence, prevalence, and mortality of disease, and the organization's own data sources, including population served, cost, high risk/high volume, and opportunity to improve, might need to be tapped to gain a sufficient understanding of the condition's potential effects on the organization's patients, enrollees, or customers. Consideration of public and company-owned data sources is essential because it cannot be assumed that data available for a general population are applicable to the specific population for whom the organization assumes responsibility.

Sociodemographic or geographic differences between the general population, for whom data is often available in the public domain, and the specific population of interest to the health care organization could be considerable. If such differences are present, the clinical condition in question might have a very different impact on the organization's population than the publicly available data would suggest. For example, cardiovascular disease continues to be the number one cause of mortality in the United States, with the disease burden being significantly associated with age. Consequently, people who are 60 years of age or older are most strongly affected. Thus, a health care organization that does not serve an older population might be considerably less interested in cardiovascular disease as a primary area of focus compared with organizations that serve a large proportion of older individuals.

In addition to a condition's prevalence and incidence, the *severity of consequences* associated with a clinical condition must also be considered. Conditions that result in only mild or moderate discomfort have different implications than conditions that are associated with serious morbidity and mortality. For example, the seriousness of upper respiratory infections (URIs) differs considerably from the sequelae associated with diabetes or HIV infection. The natural course of URI usually results in several days or weeks of discomfort and feelings of general malaise if untreated, usually followed by a full recovery. The natural course of diabetes or HIV infection, on the other hand, will result in serious morbidity, disability, and death if untreated.

Parallel to these considerations, the *organizational resources that a particular condition consumes* must also be taken into account. Conditions associated with only relatively mild symptoms may consume a seemingly disproportionate amount of resources if they are highly prevalent and if most people with the condition seek care to alleviate associated symptoms. For example, URIs can be very costly for health plans because the incidence is extremely high and individuals consume significant health care resources in alleviating discomfort. Thus, it is conceivable that an organization might spend larger amounts of resources on conditions with relatively mild or moderate morbidity, such as URIs, than on a serious condition such as HIV disease, which, on an individual basis, is much more resource intensive, but much less prevalent.

Improvability

Another concern when selecting clinical areas of focus centers around the improvability of outcomes associated with a particular condition. Two factors should be considered. First, effective interventions that significantly alter the natural course of the condition or provide palliative relief have to be available. Second, a gap must exist between the known effectiveness of the intervention and the degree to which eligible individuals receive the intervention. In other words, it needs to be determined how consistently patients receive treatments or interventions as indicated by current, state-of-the-art medical knowledge.

This gap analysis provides insight about the extent to which significant improvements are likely to be gained through focusing on a particular condition and improving associated care. Gap analysis should reflect the following considerations:

- The literature about the efficacy of appropriate interventions should be consulted. This information is often gleaned from controlled clinical trials or research using sophisticated epidemiological techniques.
- A second area of inquiry concerns the effectiveness of these interventions and the degree to which these efficacious treatments or interventions are being implemented in real world settings. If this information can be enumerated using data collected by the health care organization itself, the organization will have acquired valuable insight into its ability to translate research information into consistently delivered care. In other words, internal and external data can help identify the level of improvement that could result from closing the gap between research and real world application.
- Consideration should be given to how long it will take until the desired improved outcomes can be achieved. Some gains are likely to be immediate; others might take considerably longer. It also needs to be considered at what organizational level the targeted improvements can be put into action or who can be held responsible for achieving these improvements. In some instances, improvements are most effectively implemented by individual physicians. In other cases, larger group practices, hospitals, or health plans can implement improvements. In short, this analysis should determine who will be held responsible in the organization for the realization of improvements.
- The organization must consider what investments are necessary to make the improvements happen. Costs include direct expenses, such as investment in new technology or human resources, as well as indirect costs incurred by administering the new interventions or undertaking other associated administrative processes. Ultimately, considerations about cost-effectiveness or return on investments will need to be considered. Determining what return is sought or determining cost-effectiveness with respect to the clinical outcome can be complex.

Ultimately, monetary sums, such as how much was spent in support of the interventions, will have to be related to nonmonetary values, such as years of life gained or other outcomes that allow meaningful comparisons. At times, comparative data are sought—such as how the investment in the consistent prescription of a newly considered hyperlipidemic compares in its ability to increase years of life to other routinely applied interventions for hypertension or other conditions. Cost-effectiveness data that allow the comparison of one intervention to another are still rare and might have to be specifically performed for the conditions and interventions in question.

Customer Understanding

As health care organizations discover quality as an important competitive advantage—as manufacturing or service industries did 10 to 15 years ago—the organization's customers will come rapidly into focus. Notions of patient-centered care or continuously redesigning care processes to become more patient friendly are becoming standard business practices in innovative health care delivery organizations. This implies that the concerns and preferences of the organization's customers are being integrated into the planning and production processes. Consequently, customer input and knowledge should be considered when selecting clinical areas of focus.

Different types of health care organizations, such as clinics, hospitals, long-term facilities, managed care organizations, or integrated delivery systems, serve a variety of customers. Depending on the organizational type, customers may be consumers, purchasers, communities, care deliverers, third-party payers of health care services, or a mix of these. The interests and concerns of these customers may not completely overlap. Thus, before selecting clinical focus areas, it is wise to determine the organization's major customer groups and identify the clinical conditions that might be important to them.

The importance that various customer groups place on different clinical areas is not always driven by the most recent statistical information on disease burden, epidemiology, or cost. Clinical conditions might be considered important for a myriad of other reasons, including media attention or the fact that they are emotionally laden. For example, although mortality from lung cancer outranks mortality from breast cancer among women today, breast cancer is perceived as the more important health concern for women.

Information about customer preferences is often less available and quantifiable for health care organizations than for other industries. Gaining a meaningful understanding of customers' needs requires sophisticated market research and customer surveying that is not routine for many health care organizations. At times, anecdotal evidence and managers' gut feelings are substituted for more methodologically sound methods of inquiry for pinpointing customer preferences. The risk of misunderstanding customers is obviously much higher when using such intuitive methods than when using more quantifiable approaches.

Although not a customer in the strictest sense, regulatory bodies, such as the National Committee for Quality Assurance (NCQA) or the Joint Commission on Accreditation of Healthcare Organizations (Joint Commission), and their respective accreditation requirements should also be considered when selecting clinical focus areas. These organizations might require data collection and reporting in specific clinical areas. Ignoring these requirements when selecting clinical focus areas could result in added work that cannot be simultaneously used to satisfy regulatory requirements. An effective combination of organizational clinical priorities and regulatory requirements may lead to increased efficiencies.

Organizational Understanding

Finally, a health care organization should consider an organization-wide assessment before selecting focus areas. This assessment must address a number of questions, including the following:

- Can credible and energetic champions for specific focus areas be identified within the organization? Champions within the organization serve as catalysts for action and can drive the improvement processes forward. These champions should be highly respected clinicians within the clinical area that is being considered for organizational focus. In most cases, champions are recruited from the ranks of senior physicians and nursing staff.
- Does an organization have a history of working on particular clinical conditions? Previous involvement in improvement activities as part of interorganizational collaboration, research, or other organized efforts can provide a firm basis for further improvement activities.
- Are there existing infrastructures for particular clinical conditions, and if so, could they be used to conduct clinical quality improvements? Such infrastructures are characterized by the existence of clinical quality improvement teams, organizational awareness of the "systemness" of clinical practice, and a capacity by front line staff to use statistical methods when improving processes.

When organizations cannot fall back on existing infrastructures, a new infrastructure must be built, which is a potentially labor- and time-intensive process. In these instances, it would be wise to focus on areas in which gains could be made relatively quickly and easily.

DETERMINING RELEVANT CRITERIA AND MAKING A SELECTION

Once all potential criteria for the selection of a clinical focus area have been identified, health care organizations must determine which criteria are relevant to their environment. Preferences and criteria have to be weighed against each other to establish their importance to the organization. Typically, senior management will be charged with such an endeavor. To sort through a set of relevant criteria for the final selection process and reach a balanced and widely supportable decision, it is often easiest to use a number of decision-making tools and techniques, ranging from "command" (one person has the authority to reach decisions independent of outside input) to "consultation" (input from others is sought, with one person making a final decision) to "consensus" (using the knowledge and experience of a group, based on input from all group members).

When making complex decisions, such as identifying clinical priority areas, the consensus model is most commonly used. Consensus decision making seeks unanimous acceptance of a group decision rather than unanimous agreement of each individual group member. Group members may use a variety of techniques, including brainstorming, multivoting, and decision matrices to reach acceptance of a group decision.

Following are the steps involved in reaching unanimous acceptance of a clinical focus:

- *Identify all relevant criteria.* This brainstorming stage is characterized by the collection of a broad range of potentially relevant criteria without the immediate evaluation of their merit. This process can be conducted either by each group member proposing ideas or by individuals putting their ideas on pieces of paper that are sorted into groups on a storyboard.
- *Narrow the list.* After all possible criteria have been identified and a long and typically unwieldy list of criteria has been produced, the list will require some trimming. One method of narrowing the idea list is a process often called weighted

voting. Weighted voting provides a method for quantifying group members' divergent opinions and capturing support for the identified ideas and criteria. Typically, group members are given more votes than the identified options. For example, if 10 criteria have been identified, group members are given 15 votes that they can distribute among the options. They can give all their votes to one option or spread them out more evenly. Group members are encouraged to dispense their votes according to the relative strength of their preferences, rather than giving all votes to just one option. The purpose of this technique is to identify criteria and options that are widely supported by all group members.

- *Use a decision matrix.* Decision matrices are used to inject objectivity into the decision-making process. They allow group members to rate options against weighted criteria so that they can reach a group decision. Decision matrices are useful when evaluating a set of options and their alternatives. An a priori ranking system should be developed so that a differential rating of the options is possible. Rankings could range from 1 (not important) to 5 (extremely important).

Decision matrices can also be useful when evaluating potential clinical focus areas against criteria that previously have been deemed important by the group. For example, a clinical area considered for organizational focus could be rated against six criteria from the four knowledge areas, with each criterion being evaluated on a scale of 1 to 10. Each group member's rating would then be tabulated and averaged to determine the relative clinical focus areas being considered.

SELECTING THE RIGHT MEASUREMENT METHODS

Having a meaningful, well-designed measurement system is becoming an increasingly critical factor in an organization's success. Although the competitive advantage in America's health care environment has often been attained through aggressive pricing, some have theorized that offering high quality care at competitive prices will constitute the competitive frontier for health plans, hospitals, and clinics in mature managed care markets in the future.[6]

Several methods of achieving higher quality outcomes are currently used in health care settings to bring quality goals to reality. Yet, how will the success of these methods be measured? Measurement methods include total quality management (TQM) or continuous quality improvement (CQI) techniques, strategic performance measurements, and measurement through research.

Quality improvement concepts and methods originally developed for the manufacturing industry have received much attention in the health care industry over the last 10 years. Countless publications have addressed how the theories, concepts, and techniques associated with TQM/CQI can be applied to improve aspects of service and patient care in hospitals and clinics.[7] Evidence suggests that these applications can be effective in reducing cost by eliminating waste, reducing rework, and redesigning systems while improving corporate performance, employee relations, productivity, customer satisfaction, market share, and profitability.[8] Most important, these innovations have ensured the delivery of high quality care to patients.[9, 10]

Parallel to the introduction of these innovations at the front line of caregiving, innovations have also been made in how key performance and core processes methods are managed.[11, 12] Kaplan and Norton have convincingly argued that, like flying an airplane, successful stewardship of complex businesses and organizations requires the simultaneous monitoring of multiple gauges or dials that let the manager know how well the business is performing.[13, 14] Such measurements typically monitor several key dimensions, including clinical quality, customer experience and satisfaction, core processes and their results, finances, and economics, as well as learning and innovation.

With an increased emphasis on using quantifiable data to guide decisions about clinical care improvement, considerable confusion exists about what measurement methods and techniques should be used for what purposes.[15] This confusion may originate, in part, from the different measurement methods that key players in health care have been exposed to and feel comfortable with. Management's investment in any one measurement approach over another can lead to attempts to extend those techniques into areas for which they are not well suited. Measurement theories and techniques associated with TQM/CQI, clinical performance measurement, and scientific research are not identical and should not be used interchangeably.[16] However, these methods and techniques can be combined into an effective measurement system, enabling reliable monitoring of key health care processes and their outcomes, effective process redesign, prudent stewardship of rapid process improvements, and the pursuit of information about which care innovations might lead to improved patient health.

Chapter 8 provides a case study discussion to illustrate how one organization integrated these three measurement traditions into a comprehensive system.

CONCLUSION

Improvement of care and service with demonstrated results is a critical part of quality efforts, yet organizations continue to engage in elaborate improvement initiative without focus and with measurement systems that are ill planned, ineffective, or nonexistent. Focused improvement priorities with measurements that align with the organization's vision, mission, and strategies and that are meaningful to leaders and employees will be the most valuable to an organization committed to making real improvements.

References

1. Wennberg, J. E., and A. Gittlesohn, "Variations in Medical Care among Small Areas," *Scientific American* 246 (1982): 120–34.

2. Bunker, J. P., "Is Efficacy the Gold Standard for Quality Assessment?" *Inquiry* 25 (Spring, 1988): 51–8.

3. Institute of Medicine, *Assessing Medical Technologies* (Washington, D. C.: National Academy Press, 1985).

4. Dubinsky, M., and J. H. Ferguson, "Analysis of the National Institutes of Health Medicare Coverage Assessment," *International Journal of Technology Assessment in Health Care* 6, no. 3 (1990): 480–8.

5. Thorndike, A. N., et al., "National Patterns in the Treatment of Smokers by Physicians," *Journal of the American Medical Association* 279, no. 8 (Feb. 25, 1998): 604–8.

6. Chassin, M. R., "Assessing Strategies for Quality Improvement," *Health Affairs* 16, no. 3 (1997): 151–61.

7. Banks, N. J., et al., "Variability in Clinical Systems: Applying Modern Quality Control Methods to Health Care," *Journal on Quality Improvement* 21 no. 8 (1995): 407–19.

8. Mendelowitz, A. I., *Total Quality Management Practices*, B-243493. (Washington, D. C.: U. S. General Accounting Office, 1991): 1–42.

9. McLaughlin, C. P., and K. N. Simpson, "Does TQM/CQI Work in Health Care?" In McLaughlin, C. P., and A. D. Kaluzny, eds., *Continuous Quality Improvement in Health Care: Theory, Implementation, and Applications* (Gaithersburg, Md.: Aspen, 1994): 33–44.

10. Nelson, E. C., et al., "Report Cards or Instrument Panels: Who Needs What?" *Journal on Quality Improvement* 21, no. 4 (1995): 155–66.

11. Nelson, E. C., et al., "Improving Health Care, Part I: The Clinical Value Compass," *Journal on Quality Improvement* 22, no. 4 (1996): 243–58.

12. Ribnick, P. G., and V. A. Carrano, "Understanding the New Era in Health Care Accountability: Report Cards," *Journal of Nursing Care Quality* 10, no. 1 (1995): 1–18.

13. Kaplan, R. S., and D. P. Norton, *Translating Theory into Action: The Balanced Scorecard* (Boston: Harvard Business School Press, 1996).

14. Kaplan, R. S., and D. P. Norton, "The Balanced Scorecard— Measures That Drive Performance," *Harvard Business Review* 70, no. 1 (1992): 71–9.

15. Kaluzny, A. D., et al., "Continuous Quality Improvement in the Clinical Setting: Enhancing Adoption," *Quality Management in Health Care* 1, no. 1 (1992): 37–44.

16. Solberg, L. I., et al., "The Three Faces of Performance Measurement: Improvement, Accountability, and Research," *Journal on Quality Improvement* 23, no. 3 (1997): 135–47.

Suggested Readings

Banks, N. J., et al., "Variability in Clinical Systems: Applying Modern Quality Control Methods to Health Care," *Journal on Quality Improvement* 21, no. 8 (1995): 407–19.

Batalden, P. B., and P. K. Stoltz, "A Framework for the Continual Improvement of Health Care: Building and Applying Professional and Improvement Knowledge to Test Changes in Daily Work," *Journal on Quality Improvement* 19, no. 10 (1993): 424–52.

Batalden, P. B., et al., "Linking Outcomes Measurement to Continual Improvement: The Serial 'V' Way of Thinking about Improving Clinical Care," *Journal on Quality Improvement* 20, no. 4 (1994): 167–80.

Berwick, D. M., et al., *Curing Health Care: New Strategies for Quality Improvement* (San Francisco: Jossey-Bass, 1991).

Brailer, D. J., et al., "Physician-Led Clinical Performance Improvement: A New Model for Quality Management," *Journal of Clinical Outcomes Measurement* 4, no. 5 (1997): 33–6.

Carr, D. B., et al., *Acute Pain Management: Operative and Medical Procedures and Trauma. Clinical Practice Guidelines No. 1.* (Rockville, Md.: U. S. Department of Health and Human Services, Public Health Service, Agency for Health Care Policy and Research, AHCPR Publication No. 92-0032, 1992).

Chassin, M. R., "Assessing Strategies for Quality Improvement," *Health Affairs* 16, no. 3 (1997): 151–61.

Coddington, D. C., et al., *Making Integrated Health Care Work* (Englewood, Colo.: Center for Research in Ambulatory Health Care Administration, 1996).

Fiore, M. C., et al., *Smoking Cessation. Clinical Practice Guidelines No. 18* (Rockville, Md.: U. S. Department of Health and Human Services, Public Health Service, Agency for Health Care Policy and Research, AHCPR Publication No. 96-0692, 1996).

Genovich-Richards, J., "The Customer: Perspectives and Expectations of Quality." In Meisenheimer, C. G., ed., *Improving Quality: A Guide to Effective Programs* (Gaithersburg, Md.: Aspen, 1997): 133–46.

Hibbard, J. H., and J. J. Jewett, "Will Quality Report Cards Help Consumers?" *Health Affairs* 16, no. 3 (1997): 218–28.

James, B. C., "Implementing Practice Guidelines through Clinical Quality Improvement," *Frontiers of Health Services Management* 10, no. 1 (1993): 3–37.

Joint Commission on Accreditation of Healthcare Organizations, *Manual for Hospitals* (Chicago: The Joint Commission, 1992).

Kaluzny, A. D., et al., "Continuous Quality Improvement in the Clinical Setting: Enhancing Adoption," *Quality Management in Health Care* 1, no. 1 (1992): 37–44.

Kaplan, R. S., and D. P. Norton, The Balanced Scorecard—Measures That Drive Performance," *Harvard Business Review* 70, no. 1 (1992): 71–9.

Kaplan, R. S., and D. P. Norton, *Translating Theory into Action: The Balanced Scorecard* (Boston: Harvard Business School Press, 1996).

Kongstvedt, P. R., "Using Data in Medical Management." In Kongstvedt, P., ed., *Essentials of Managed Healthcare,* 2d edition (Gaithersburg, Md.: Aspen, 1997): 312–24.

McLaughlin, C. P., and A. D. Kaluzny, "Managing with TQM in a Professional Organization." In McLaughlin C. P., and A. D. Kaluzny, eds., *Continuous Quality Improvement in Health Care: Theory, Implementation, and Applications* (Gaithersburg, Md.: Aspen, 1994): 187–97.

McLaughlin, C. P., and K. N. Simpson, "Does TQM/CQI Work in Health Care?" In McLaughlin C. P., and A. D. Kaluzny, eds., *Continuous Quality Improvement in Health Care: Theory, Implementation, and Applications* (Gaithersburg, Md.: Aspen, 1994): 33–44.

Mendelowitz, A. I., *Total Quality Management Practices,* B-243493 (Washington, D. C.: U. S. General Accounting Office, 1991): 1–42.

National Committee on Quality Assurance, *Standards for the Accreditation of Managed Care Organizations,* 3d edition (Washington, D. C.: National Committee on Quality Assurance, 1996).

Nelson, E. C., et al., "Improving Health Care, Part I: The Clinical Value Compass" *Journal on Quality Improvement* 22, no. 4 (1996): 243–58.

Nelson, E. C., et al., "Report Cards or Instrument Panels: Who Needs What?" *Journal on Quality Improvement* 21, no. 4 (1995): 155–66.

Ribnick, P. G., and V. A. Carrano, "Understanding the New Era in Health Care Accountability: Report Cards," *Journal of Nursing Care Quality* 10, no. 1 (1995): 1–18.

Rooney, E., "TQM/CQI in Business and Health Care: An Overview," *American Association of Occupational Health Nurses Journal* 40, no. 7 (1992): 319–25.

Rosner, B., *Fundamentals of Biostatistics* (Boston, Mass.: PWS-Kent, 1990).

Schoenbaum, S. C., et al., *Using Clinical Practice Guidelines to Evaluate Quality of Care* (U. S. Department of Health and Human Services, Public Health Service, Agency for Health Care Policy and Research, AHCPR Publication No. 95-0045/46, 1995).

Shortell, S. M., et al., *Remaking Health Care in America: Building Organized Delivery Systems* (San Francisco: Jossey-Bass, 1996).

Solberg, L. I., et al., "The three faces of performance measurement: improvement, accountability, and research," *Journal on Quality Improvement* 23, no. 3 (1997): 135–47.

VanAmringe, M., and T. E. Shannon, "Awareness, Assimilation, and Adoption: The Challenge of Effective Dissemination and the First AHCPR-Sponsored Guidelines," *Quality Review Bulletin* 18, no.12 (1992): 397–404.

Wennberg, J. E., and A. Gittlesohn, "Variations in Medical Care among Small Areas," *Scientific American* 246 (1982): 120–34.

8

Building an Integrated Quality Measurement and Improvement System

Joachim Roski, PhD
Julianne M. Morath

To maximize clinical quality improvements, Allina Health System (AHS) decided to focus on just a few, high leverage clinical areas. Five priority conditions were determined through careful analysis, taking into account disease burden, high cost/volume, and identifiable opportunities for improvement. It was believed that health conditions meeting these criteria could demonstrate the "value-added" benefits of providing care in a vertically integrated health system. The result of this analysis led AHS to select pregnancy, diabetes, cardiovascular disease (CV) or acute myocardial infarction (AMI), pediatric asthma, and oncology (breast or colon cancer).

This chapter illustrates how AHS integrated three measurement traditions into a comprehensive system to demonstrate performance, enable improvement at the front line, and carefully study innovations. AHS's system allows the organization to measure performance, improvement, and research. The purpose, structure, and implementation of these measurement components are outlined in addition to how the components are interconnected.

PERFORMANCE MEASUREMENT

A primary objective of AHS's measurement system is to provide information about the consistent delivery and improvement of clinical care quality. AHS is pursuing the following question under its

149

clinical performance measurement strategy: Are we doing what we know we should be doing? The organization's pursuit of the answer to this question is critical because the occurrence of problems in the overuse, underuse, or misuse of care procedures among caregivers has been convincingly demonstrated.[1]

Identifying Best Practices

Before pursuing an answer to the preceding question, a number of issues require resolution. Initially, the "what we know we should be doing" needs to be established through careful review of the evidence concerning the efficacy, effectiveness, and cost-effectiveness of relevant care processes. On a national level, a number of organizations and expert groups have begun to identify what constitutes best practice. These include government organizations, such as the Agency for Health Care Policy and Research; professional organizations, such as the American Medical Association and its sections; and local health plans, medical groups, and hospitals.

Ideally, identified care recommendations should be based on sound evidence. When evidence is nonexistent or equivocal, expert consensus should be sought. To be effectively used in any particular care setting, these best practices—also called pathways, care standards, or guidelines—often need to be adapted to local conditions.[2] Once best practices have been made explicit, they need to be put into practice, and the degree of implementation success should be captured by measuring progress.

Structuring Performance Measures

AHS's clinical performance measurement efforts are part of its overall performance measurement strategy. In addition to clinical care excellence, measures of customer experience and satisfaction, growth, internal work environment, and economic performance have been identified. Measurements for all five of AHS's prioritized clinical conditions have been developed to determine to what degree superior clinical care excellence is apparent throughout the system, as evidenced by current research. The following examples of clinical performance measures were designed to capture a number of important aspects of organizational performance:

- Measurement panels reflecting care issues across the continuum of care were constructed for all prioritized conditions. This seemed particularly appropriate for the complexities of a vertically integrated health system because all of the prioritized conditions require that care be delivered in multiple settings and clinical episodes can last for many months.

- Measures on process and outcomes of clinical care, customer satisfaction with care, and the economic impact of delivering and improving care were captured.
- The organizational level that should be held responsible for the improvement of these measures was determined. Therefore, system-wide rates and clinically and methodologically defensible rates at the lowest sensible aggregation level, such as health plan product, hospital, medical group, and clinic, are calculated.

Continuous quality improvement/total quality management (CQI/TQM) theory posits that substandard outputs are caused by suboptimal system design rather than the failure of individuals operating within that system. Thus, substandard outputs are most effectively improved by analyzing system-level data rather than by identifying a few individuals performing well below standard within that system.[3] Therefore, although creating practice profiles of individual physicians is considered important in medical and network management,[4] providing "system-level" (hospital, medical group, clinic) data feedback might be preferable to continuously and systematically foster improvements because such data reflects that care is provided in the context of a care team and care setting. In addition, it is often difficult to obtain large enough samples at the individual provider level to reliably represent individual practice patterns of interest.[5, 6]

Figure 8-1 illustrates the blueprint for AHS's clinical performance measurement system architecture. It shows how the clinical care excellence measurements for its prioritized clinical conditions are a subset of AHS's overall performance measurement system, how measures are identified along the continuum of care, and how AHS-wide rates are comprised of rates at the lowest level of aggregation.

Engaging Clinicians in Performance Measurement

Because AHS considered it futile to build a measurement system that clinicians fundamentally disagreed with in terms of its purpose, structure, or chosen measures, it seemed important to build a system with measures that clinicians would regard as clinically meaningful and that were supported by valid data. Clinicians had

FIGURE 8-1.   Overview of AHS's Clinical Performance
Measurement System

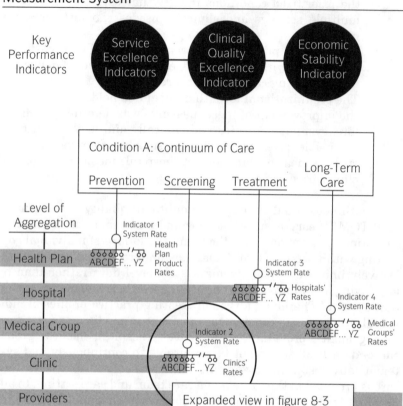

Reprinted, with permission, from Allina Health System, Minnetonka, Minn., 1998.

had bad experiences with past measurement efforts based on data
they either considered invalid or not representative of their practice
patterns, which resulted in adverse financial consequences. At the
same time, many clinicians had limited experience with measurement theory, measurement requirements, and data collection. Thus,
it has been a primary objective to engage clinicians and other health
care professionals in the construction of AHS's clinical performance
measurement system and to create relevant measures that would
broaden clinicians' understanding of care parameters and the validity of their outcomes.

The following sections discuss ways in which the clinicians were
engaged.

Provider Groups Were Convened AHS convened community-based health care professionals who were considered experts and opinion-leaders for each of the prioritized health care conditions. These clinicians were charged with identifying community standards of care, opportunities for improvement, and promising initiatives to address existing gaps. They were also asked to oversee the implementation of key improvement tactics and projects. The organization placed improvement of clinical care and patient outcomes—not cost reduction—at the center of all these activities.[7, 8] Ultimately, however, improving clinical quality may result in cost-savings through the elimination of unintended clinical variation, process redesign that creates increased efficiency, and the consistent promotion of effective care processes.[9]

In addition, these experts were asked to contribute to AHS's clinical performance measurement system. Clinicians were very responsive to AHS's invitation to define care excellence and to identify areas in which significant improvements could be made in patient health outcomes. However, AHS's measurement agenda was greeted with a significant level of suspicion and mistrust. In particular, clinicians feared that AHS would determine what measures should be selected, how they would be put into operation, and how they would be used by clinical administrators in relative isolation from practicing clinicians. Thus, AHS's objective was to build positive relationships with participating community-based clinicians to slowly overcome their suspicion and earn their trust so that improvement would result.

Potential Measures Were Identified From the beginning, key quality staff members attended clinician meetings to understand the concerns providers had regarding their clinical measurement needs. As a first exercise in that endeavor, clinicians were asked to identify clinical measures that were of particular interest to providers. To facilitate this process, quality staff members identified dozens of measures used by researchers, regulators (the National Committee for Quality Assurance [NCQA], the Joint Commission on Accreditation of Healthcare Organizations [Joint Commission], and the state health department), local competing health care organizations, and other health care organizations around the country. In addition, quality staff formulated additional potential measures that reflected the group's ongoing discussions about clinical care excellence and its improvement. These measures were divided by type: preventive care related (early detection and screening, treatment), long-term (follow-up care) care processes, and results of care.

A Measure Set Was Selected   Subsequently, clinicians were asked to select the measures they considered the most important and relevant clinically. They were given multiple votes and were instructed to spread their votes along the continuum of care, considering both process and patient-referenced outcomes. The actual voting occurred when clinicians placed stickers onto a ballot poster that listed all identified potential measurements for a clinical condition. Making the vote public allowed clinicians to see what care aspect measures gathered the most support and interest. This procedure allowed AHS to demonstrate that the measures were neither represented by the interests of a clinician minority, nor were they selected by AHS in isolation of the input of community-based clinicians. AHS's quality staff tabulated the votes and reviewed the selected measures against measures that needed to be compiled for regulatory purposes, those in use by other health care organizations in the same market, and those formulated by the state health department. Quality staff members then presented a modified indicator list, aligned with AHS's organizational measurement interests, to the physician groups for approval. Measures of patient experience and economic impact were included in all indicator sets.

Putting Performance Measures into Operation

AHS's quality staff, in cooperation with clinician leaders, then began to put the selected measures into operation by specifying data sources used, as well as denominator(s) and nominator(s) reported for each indicator.[10] Subsequent data reports were released to the respective physician expert groups for each of Allina's prioritized clinical conditions. Clinicians were then able to identify the strengths and limitations of the indicators they had chosen. They realized that not all the measures they had chosen were useful for ongoing monitoring, either because the measure itself was ill-defined or did not focus on what the providers wanted to know or because of information system limitations. A measure that cannot be applied to drive improvement in relevant areas of practice of concern is not useful. Continuing to generate such measures is wasteful. Clinicians were then prompted to revise the selected measures, taking into consideration the following factors:

- Clinical importance
- Relevance to caregivers
- Alignment with prioritized system-wide clinical initiatives
- AHS's ability to influence the indicator

- The ability to quantify predicted changes
- Definitions of normative ranges and targets
- The ability to clearly assign accountability for the improvement of the measure
- The ability to identify extraneous influences on the measures and statistically control for them (risk adjustment)
- The availability of explicit care criteria for process measures
- Reliability and validity
- The feasibility of data collection strategies

This formative process has led to the adoption of a revised clinical performance indicator set for ongoing monitoring of each clinical condition. Figure 8-2 presents AHS's clinical performance indicator set for CV/AMI as an illustration of how their condition-specific indicator sets span the continuum of care, include process and outcome measures, and capture consumer satisfaction and economic impact. Chosen aggregation levels and the data sources that fed individual indicators are also listed.

Reporting Performance Measures to Organizational Audiences

Clinical performance measures also are reported to the Quality Committee of AHS's Board of Directors and AHS's senior management. The responsibilities of the Quality Committee include ensuring that appropriate measures are used, that feedback is provided to front line clinicians, and that improvements are reviewed in due time for units that have previously performed below target. AHS's Board of Directors has delegated responsibility for quality and performance oversight to AHS's Quality Committee. Regular reports are furnished to AHS's Board of Directors at the discretion of the Quality Committee and upon board request.

Senior management uses clinical performance measures to determine company direction and identify corrections in the course of their work. AHS's clinical performance indicator panels have created a new process and customer consciousness at the system and local levels. The panels have allowed senior managers to gather intelligence about the company's core products—care and service—and have created the impetus to ensure that local changes are consistently and continuously being implemented to enhance performance. Data presentations that plot actual performance against identified best-in-class targets have focused management's ability to identify these gaps and make the investments required to close them.

FIGURE 8-2. AHS's Clinical Performance Indicator Set for CV/AMI

No.	Indicator	Level of Aggregation	Data Source
1	Rate of patients with AMI who are admitted to a hospital (stratified by age and gender)	Health plan products	Health plan administrative claims
2	Time from onset of chest pain to arrival at hospital for medical evaluation	Hospitals	Hospital patient records
3	On-scene time of emergency transportation services	Transportation services	Transportation service administration records
4	Time from admission to emergency department to receiving (a) thrombolytic therapy (b) angioplasty	Hospitals	Hospital patient records
5	Rate of eligible patients who receive a prescription for β-blockers at time of discharge from hospital	Hospitals	Health plan administrative claims
6	Rate of eligible patients who receive smoking cessation advice/counseling during/following hospitalization	Hospitals	Hospital patient records
7	Rate of patients expressing complete satisfaction with overall care at discharge/6 months/12 months after discharge	Hospitals	Patient survey
8	Functional status at discharge/6 months/12 months	Hospitals	Patient survey
9	Mortality rate ≤30, ≤60, and ≤180 days of hospital admission	Hospitals/clinics	Health plan administrative claims, death certificates
10	Average cost per patient	Health plan products; hospitals/clinics	Health plan administrative data; hospital administrative data

Reprinted, with permission, from Allina Health System, Minnetonka, Minn., 1998.

MEASUREMENT FOR IMPROVEMENT

The use of CQI/TQM's principles, methodologies, and techniques in American health care settings has been widespread since the mid-1980s.[11, 12] Rising health care costs are a major societal concern, and with the arrival of prepaid health services, cost containment has become a major business priority for all health care delivery organizations. CQI/TQM analyzes production processes to identify unintended variation and, ultimately, identify opportunities for reducing cost. To successfully engage in meaningful continuous improvement efforts, organizations need to acquire a deep understanding of systems, variation, work and organizational psychology, and the theory of knowledge.[13] Because virtually all clinical processes involve many stakeholders, such as physicians, nurses, lab technicians, pharmacists, and administrative staff, it is essential to create cross-functional work teams of these stakeholders for effective process improvement. These work teams guarantee that all individuals involved in the process can analyze their segment of the "production" process and assume ownership and responsibility for keeping it strong and successful. Statistical approaches such as time plots, run charts, and scatter diagrams are used to understand the causes of variation and the effectiveness of improvement activities.

Using the PDSA Cycle

Although the specific measurement techniques supporting improvement are customized at the local level in AHS's individual care delivery units and health plans, the underlying structure of improvement processes is identical. Once a problem has been identified (for example, through performance measurement), an improvement team strives to answer three basic questions and to build a measurement system that helps answer them:

1. What are we trying to accomplish?
2. How will we know that a change is an improvement?
3. What changes can we make that we predict will lead to improvement?[14]

Local cross-functional improvement teams engage in *p*lanning, *d*oing, *s*tudying, and *a*cting activities to find the answers to these three questions. Activity cycles based on these activities are also known as *PDSA* cycles.[15] The ongoing evaluation of improvement activities that are part of the PDSA cycle involves measures that are typically based on small samples. These "rough" or "good enough" measures are more practical than the rigorous measurements associated with research that often are not feasible to adopt.

Linking Performance Measurement to Improvement

AHS's performance measures provide regular snapshots of the entire system, allowing units to compare their ability to reach identified targets and letting managers decide whether additional organizational resources are needed to reach performance targets at local sites. Although the degree of suboptimal outcomes at different sites might be similar, the cause for these outcomes and likely strategies to improve on them might differ substantially among sites. If suboptimal outcomes are detected through centrally conducted clinical performance measurements, locally developed process improvement strategies can be implemented to affect those undesired outcomes. Measurement techniques associated with CQI/TQM are then used to continually evaluate the improvement strategies for their feasibility and effectiveness. Effective stewardship of resources is monitored by defining milestones in the improvement process and setting target dates by which milestones are expected to be reached. Figure 8-3 illustrates the interface of clinical performance measurement and process improvement. The CQI/TQM process, including a PDSA cycle, is graphically represented.

For example, at AHS, customer feedback data and provider experience signaled a need to examine performance in inpatient pain management. The data revealed variability in physician-prescribed pharmaceuticals, nurse assessment, and response times to patient reports of pain. Patterns of dissatisfaction by patients in their experience of pain management were also revealed. This evidence sparked a system-wide initiative to undertake local improvements.

Acute pain management guidelines[16] were selected for implementation in various hospitals. One site was identified to pilot the implementation. A cross-functional task force was identified for design and measurement of this initiative. Levers for accelerating change, such as standardizing orders for pain medication, were identified, and a PDSA cycle was set in motion. Regular progress reports on the pilot process, milestones achieved, and results being realized were provided to clinical leaders throughout the system. Information gained through the pilot was then used to foster rapid implementation in other hospitals using similar local cross-functional teams, process redesign, PDSA cycles, and associated measurement techniques.

FIGURE 8-3. How Measurement for Improvement Relates to
Performance Measurement

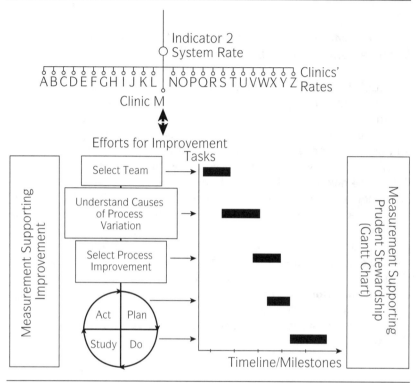

Reprinted, with permission, from Allina Health System, Minnetonka, Minn., 1998.

MEASUREMENT FOR RESEARCH

Innovation in patient care has traditionally used evidence gained in
randomized research trials that compare promising new treatments
and interventions to one or more alternatives. The methods associated with this approach are rigorous and can eliminate the possibility that the difference between the examined innovation and its
alternative can be attributed to anything but the intervention in
question. New interventions are accepted or rejected as superior to
the alternative with a predetermined statistical likelihood of
error. Complex statistical techniques based on a set of assumptions
rooted in probability theory are crucial aids in that process. Alpha-
and beta-errors, confidence intervals, means and standard devia-
tions, multivariate analyses of variance, odds ratios, dependent and

independent variables, and covariance are terms closely related to the research approach to measurement.[17]

Research Measurement Compared with Performance and Improvement Measurement

Although many aspects of research are clearly appealing—statistical theory and the rigorous measurement procedures, for example—the unreflected adoption of research as the primary measurement method is impractical and inappropriate. Research, performance, and improvement measurements all have different purposes.[18]

Whereas measurement associated with research tries to establish new knowledge about what care or intervention should be applied, performance measurement tries to establish how consistently the new knowledge can be translated into practice. Process improvement uses concrete, local process changes to close identified gaps in the provision of optimal care. Or, to put it simply, research measurement pursues the question: What care should we give patients with a particular condition? Performance measurement pursues the question: Are we giving the care we know we should be giving to patients with a particular condition? And CQI/TQM asks: How can we improve our local processes to give patients with a particular condition the care we know we should be giving?

Research in Health Care Organizations

The pursuit of knowledge about appropriate patient care innovations is mostly pursued by academic medical centers and research laboratories funded by public sources, such as the National Institutes of Health, and private sources such as pharmaceutical companies. An increasing number of health care organizations have also built important research centers, such as Group Health Cooperative Puget Sound and Kaiser Permanente.

AHS uses a research measurement framework when investigating promising care approaches that have unknown effectiveness. For example, although the efficacy of physician advice to quit smoking has been demonstrated, the effectiveness of the complete implementation of the Agency for Health Care Policy and Research's smoking cessation guidelines has not been unequivocally demonstrated.[19] Because tobacco control is one of AHS's premier health improvement goals, a quasi-experimental research study randomizing 20 Allina-owned clinics to 2 experimental conditions was initiated to investigate the impact of the implementation of these guidelines on practice patterns and patient cessation rates. Rigorous adherence to scientific measurement theory and criteria was observed to test the impact of the implementation. At the conclusion of this study, recommendations regarding the system-wide implementation of all aspects of these guidelines are expected.

The measurement scope of this project exceeds the requirements of the CQI/TQM framework by far. For example, to satisfy experimental design and measurement concerns, more than 2,000 patient surveys were collected for each clinic enrolled in the study. This data volume and its associated costs differ substantially from measurement associated with CQI/TQM efforts.

CONCLUSION

AHS's concentration on data-driven decision making has led to the creation of a measurement system that incorporates methods from strategic performance measurement, measurement for improvement (CQI), and research. A careful evaluation of the appropriateness and utility of these measurement paradigms has allowed AHS to use measurement techniques in three traditions: performance measurement, CQI/TQM, and research. The example of AHS is germane to understanding the role of measurement in evidenced-based decision making, improvement, and innovation.

Measurement of identified core processes and their improvement has focused AHS's management team on those processes. Although clinical performance measures have been successfully used for internal purposes, AHS has not tested these measures to determine whether they might also be perceived as helpful by consumers and purchasers of health care. In general, consumer preferences on clinical quality are not very well understood.[20] Furthermore, consumers and purchasers will be able to compare competing health care organizations' ability to deliver clinical quality only if these organizations use identical data collection and analysis procedures.

AHS's measurement system is contributing to its overall organizational ability to manage knowledge, a fundamental concept of quality and a skill that is integral to a successful, mature, vertically integrated health care system.[21] Such a system is characterized by the collection of information on the health needs of consumers and communities; an understanding of resource needs across the continuum of care; an understanding of the caregiving processes that promote, enhance, maintain, and restore health in a cost-effective manner; knowledge of what the system knows and what the system doesn't know; the ability to quickly improve processes under changing circumstances; the consistent fulfillment of stakeholder expectations; and an investment in human capital.

References

1. Brailer, D. J., et al., "Physician-Led Clinical Performance Improvement: A New Model for Quality Management," *Journal of Clinical Outcomes Measurement* 4, no. 5 (1997): 33–6.

2. Coddington, D. C., et al., *Making Integrated Health Care Work* (Englewood, Colo.: Center for Research in Ambulatory Health Care Administration, 1996).

3. McLaughlin, C. P., and K. N. Simpson, "Does TQM/CQI work in health care?" In McLaughlin, C. P., and A. D. Kaluzny, eds., *Continuous Quality Improvement in Health Care: Theory, Implementation, and Applications* (Gaithersburg, Md.: Aspen, 1994): 33–44.

4. Wennberg, J. E., and A. Gittlesohn, "Variations in Medical Care among Small Areas," *Scientific American* 246 (1982): 120–34.

5. VanAmringe, M., and T. E. Shannon, "Awareness, Assimilation, and Adoption: The Challenge of Effective Dissemination and the First AHCPR-Sponsored Guidelines," *Quality Review Bulletin* 18, no. 12 (1992): 397–404.

6. McLaughlin, C. P., and A. D. Kaluzny, "Managing with TQM in a Professional Organization." In McLaughlin, C. P., and A. D. Kaluzny, eds., *Continuous Quality Improvement in Health Care: Theory, Implementation, and Applications* (Gaithersburg, Md.: Aspen, 1994): 187–97.

7. Kongstvedt, P. R., "Using Data in Medical Management." In Kongstvedt, P., ed., *Essentials of Managed Health Care*, 2d edition (Gaithersburg, Md.: Aspen, 1997): 312–24.

8. Kongstvedt, pp. 312–24.

9. Solberg, L. I., et al., "The Three Faces of Performance Measurement: Improvement, Accountability, and Research," *Journal on Quality Improvement* 23, no. 3 (1997): 135–47.

10. Schoenbaum, S. C., et al., *Using Clinical Practice Guidelines to Evaluate Quality of Care* (Rockville, Md.: U. S. Department of Health and Human Services, Public Health Service, Agency for Health Care Policy and Research, AHCPR Publication No. 95-0045/46, 1995).

11. Berwick, D. M., et al., *Curing Health Care: New Strategies for Quality Improvement* (San Francisco: Jossey-Bass, 1991).

12. Rooney, E., "TQM/CQI in Business and Health Care: An Overview," *American Association of Occupational Health Nurses Journal* 40, no. 7 (1992): 319–25.

13. Batalden, P. B., and P. K. Stoltz, "A Framework for the Continual Improvement of Health Care: Building and Applying Professional and Improvement Knowledge to Test Changes in Daily Work," *Journal on Quality Improvement* 19, no. 10 (1993): 424–52.

14. Batalden and Stoltz, pp. 424–52.

15. Batalden, P. B., et al., "Linking Outcomes Measurement to Continual Improvement: The Serial 'V' Way of Thinking about Improving Clinical Care," *Journal on Quality Improvement* 20, no. 4 (1994): 167–80.

16. Carr, D. B., et al., *Acute Pain Management: Operative and Medical Procedures and Trauma. Clinical Practice Guidelines No. 1* (Rockville, Md.: U. S. Department of Health and Human Services, Public Health Service, Agency for Health Care Policy and Research, AHCPR Publication No. 92-0032, 1992).

17. Rosner, B., *Fundamentals of Biostatistics* (Boston: PWS-Kent, 1990).

18. Solberg, et al., pp. 135–47.

19. Fiore, M. C., et al., *Smoking Cessation. Clinical Practice Guidelines No. 18* (Rockville, Md.: U. S. Department of Health and Human Services, Public Health Service, Agency for Health Care Policy and Research, AHCPR Publication No. 96-0692, 1996).

20. Hibbard, J. H., and J. J. Jewett, "Will Quality Report Cards Help Consumers?" *Health Affairs* 16, no. 3 (1997): 218–28.

21. Shortell, S. M., et al., *Remaking Health Care in America: Building Organized Delivery Systems* (San Francisco: Jossey-Bass, 1996).

Suggested Readings

"Evaluating and Using Report Cards," *Journal on Quality Improvement Joint Commission on Accreditation of Healthcare Organizations* 24, no. 1 (Jan., 1998).

Bushick, B., "Performance Indicators for Achieving Goals at Allina," *Quality Letter* 8, no. 5 (June, 1996).

Carey, R. G., and R. C. Lloyd, *Measuring Quality Improvement in Healthcare* (New York: Quality Resources, 1995).

James, B. C., "Good Enough? Standards and Measurement in Continuous Quality Improvement." In *Bridging the Gap Between Theory and Practice* (Chicago: Hospital Research and Education Trust, American Hospital Association, 1992).

Kaplan, R. S., *The Balanced Scorecard: Translating Strategy into Action* (Boston: Harvard Business School Press, 1996).

Langley, G. J., et al., *The Improvement Guide: A Practical Approach to Enhancing Organizational Performance* (San Francisco: Jossey-Bass, 1996).

Langley, G. J., Nolan, and Nolan, "The Foundation of Improvement," *Quality Progress* 27, no. 6 (June 1, 1994).

Measuring Corporate Performance, *Harvard Business Review* (Cambridge, Mass.: Harvard Business Press, 1997).

Nelson, E. C., P. Batalden, et al., "Report Cards or Instrument Panels: Who Needs What?" *Journal of Quality Improvement Joint Commission on Accreditation of Healthcare Organizations* 21, no. 4 (1995): 155–66.

Wheeler, D., *Understanding Variation* (Knoxville: SPC Press, 1993).

9

Using Measures for Performance Management

Joachim Roski, PhD

An organization that fosters curiosity, continuous learning, and widely shared responsibility for improving system performance, rather than for identifying a few outlying "bad" individual performers on whom organizational woes can be blamed and who will "need to be brought in line," can move beyond a defensive, blaming stand to a proactive position in managing performance. An organization's performance can be guided, improved, and propelled by the effective and appropriate use of data. At the same time, performance can be undermined, side-tracked, and sabotaged by counterproductive techniques that mismanage performance indicators. Mismanaging the use of organizational performance data about core processes and their impact on patient's health and well-being, satisfaction, and bottom line represents a substantial risk to an organization's success.

This chapter explores the opportunities for and barriers to effective performance management using three characteristics of quality-focused organizations: recognition that value includes both high quality and competitive price, the need to continuously strive for improvements in efficiency and outcomes, and the need to create an organizational environment that fosters trust and minimizes fear among its employees and physicians. The chapter also discusses the ways in which leaders can effectively manage performance data and the specific responsibilities of different organizational players with respect to performance data management.

CHARACTERISTICS OF ORGANIZATIONS COMMITTED TO QUALITY

A number of theorists and practitioners, including Deming, Juran, Baldrige, and Senge, have identified organizational characteristics that are key to building an organizational culture that fosters learning, that can identify methods of improving work process efficiency, that is committed to improving outcomes, and that consistently exceeds key customer expectations. An organization that is built on such characteristics differs sharply from a hierarchical, authority-satisfying, task-focused organization.

Although they individually emphasize slightly different aspects of achieving high quality processes and outputs, a number of common themes emerge. The three following themes are used to illustrate to what extent data-based management can affect these characteristics:

1. It's value not cost.
2. Improvement is never finished.
3. Create trust—eliminate fear.

It's Value not Cost

Health care organizations have focused for years on eliminating cost and waste from their production processes. This focus is particularly warranted for organizations that are financially at risk for the services they perform. Thus, the more experience health care organizations have gained in assuming risk for their patients or health consumers, the more motivated and experienced they are at reducing unintended variations in practice patterns and eliminating inefficiencies, rework, and unnecessary services. Managed care organizations, hospitals, and clinics that operate in mature managed care markets—those with most of the population in managed care, with only a few managed care organizations in the market, and with a high proportion of providers who share risk—tend to be most experienced in reducing inefficiencies. California and the Twin Cities (Minneapolis–St. Paul, Minnesota) currently represent such mature markets.

In the most advanced markets, price competition between organizations has reached the financial bottom, with organizations realizing that they cannot lower their prices any further. The next competitive frontier in these markets is the ability to offer customers "value"—superior product at the lowest possible price—as opposed to low cost only. Product value for health care organizations is determined by a number of dimensions, including superior clinical outcomes, functional status, satisfaction with care experiences, decreased morbidity and mortality, and cost-efficiencies. These measurements of value and organizational performance must be recognized by the organization's data collection, analysis, and data-based management techniques. Ideally, the organization should develop a system of measurements that reflects these aspects of value at every level of the organization—superior, patient-focused outcomes in the clinical service and economic areas.

Recognizing the Dimensions of Performance   Data-based performance management represents an opportunity for a health care organization to recognize and reinforce the dimensions of performance at all levels of the organization. The organization and its units should be held accountable for more than just making a difference within one value dimension such as the bottom line. Instead, efforts made to delight health care consumers and purchasers with superior clinical and service quality must also be rewarded. Being held accountable to the dimensions of performance represents a significant departure for professionals in traditional health care organizations. It may be a significant change for physicians to be held accountable for their ability to meet patient expectations for receiving information and education in an understandable manner, for clinical services that are provided seamlessly, and for an overall satisfactory care experience. Similarly, administrators might be unaccustomed to being held accountable for meeting the needs and expectations of external customers such as patients and purchasers and internal customers such as staff clinicians. These needs include the ability to create simple and transparent intake, discharge, billing, or approval procedures and processes. They also include providing administrative support for reorganizing inefficient work processes, organizing and providing pertinent on-the-job training and education, and ensuring that critical clinical information is provided in time. Focusing measures in the area of utilization and cost alone risks the alienation of clinicians who tend to be less interested in the economic correlates of care than in ensuring improvements in clinical and service quality for patients under their care.

It is true that "what we measure receives attention." Therefore, measures that reflect the many dimensions of performance reinforce the idea that simultaneous improvement of clinical, service, and economic outcomes is increasingly important to attract and satisfy customers in the health care industry.

Improvement Is Never Finished

One key quality theory is that quality can always be improved upon; quality never reaches a plateau that cannot be overcome to reach even higher levels. Continuous quality improvement and total quality management theories contend that quality improvement is an ongoing organizational process.

Recognizing the Dimensions of Performance Using data-based management can either enforce or undermine this notion in several critical ways:

- Selecting critical indicators that represent the organization's key strategic initiatives keeps the strategy real, simple, and out in front of employees. Ideally, well-chosen organizational performance indicators are a concrete example of organizational strategies. These indicators provide the organization with the chance to share their strategies with all layers of the organization, including those employees at the front line. Performance indicators that represent organizational intent will be used as gauges of the organization's ability to execute against its identified strategies to reach desired results. This is analogous to using the gauges of the car—speed, fuel, compass—to determine the capacity to reach a determined destination. Measures that do not closely mirror strategy are doomed to fail because they do not advance organizational aims. These measures will quickly be regarded as expendable or even wasteful to produce and review.
- Effective management of performance data helps the health care organization identify areas that need improvement. This is significantly aided by the determination of performance targets or the benchmarks that provide an illustration of what is possible. By identifying these targets, the organization and its managers can assess their performance against those who are best-in-class. Targets allow all levels of the organization to identify the gap between the current and the desired organizational performances and to mobilize the organizational energy needed to close that gap.
- Taking frequent measures over time allows managers and other employees to determine whether new investments and efforts are closing the gap between the current and desired state of organizational performance. Infrequent measurement of organizational performance is a significant barrier to the organization's ability to evaluate whether current in-

vestments in changed work processes or other improvement efforts appear to be paying off in the interim.

- Another opportunity to foster continuous improvement comes with the inclusion of performance targets into the incentive and reward structure of operational, management, and front-line teams. Expecting improvement from performance measures as part of an employee's professional responsibilities can be an additional motivational impetus to close the gap between reality and the desired organizational state. This tactic stresses the notion of professional accountability for specific, measurable, and tangible goals rather than the individual professional autonomy which, until recently, has dominated health care delivery. In the past, health care professionals—including physicians—rarely received incentives based on their ability to improve clinical outcomes or provide service experiences or on the degree to which they contributed to the bottom line. Organizations that opt not to invest in data-based management risk losing the ability to identify performance trends and problems before they reach crisis status and hamper the organization's ability to collectively improve work.

Create Trust—Eliminate Fear

Being unafraid to risk innovation and test promising ideas is one of the cornerstones of a learning organization, a theme expressed throughout this book. The ability to develop and nurture an organizational culture of inquiry is an important way of ensuring that all employees have the potential to develop and contribute to their fullest. Employees will be hesitant if the risk for failure is severe. Fear and mistrust of potential innovations are anathema to organizations committed to improving quality.

Recognizing the Dimensions of Performance   Data-based management is a chance to create and foster trust and cooperation. On the other hand, it can become a major impediment to creating an organizational environment that supports continuous improvements and innovation. Will data be used in a manner that fosters constructive dialogue and inquiry, free of blaming individuals, or will it be used to identify individuals or groups who are performing below expectation so that they can suffer the consequences for their substandard performance?

A negative, sanctioning environment can be a significant barrier for effective, data-based management. That kind of environment may invite employees to play games with the measurement system. It may also create perverse incentives for performing well on performance standards that lead to unexpected side effects. These phenomena can take several forms. Playing games with the measurement system can occur if employees feel compelled to manipulate data collection or analysis they believe will be used to hurt them. This risk increases with the level of control that employees have over data elements that feed into the indicators. This risk is also proportional to the degree that individuals fear and expect negative consequences based on performance data. The risk is minimized if managers and other employees feel invested in the indicators themselves and see them as valuable to the organization's performance and to patients' health. To accept performance indicators, employees need input into the creation of the indicators. This input can ensure that employees feel committed to improving performance and can help adopt the kind of quantifiable performance measures that are essential to true improvement.

Another barrier to improvement is the degree to which measuring certain performance indicators creates perverse incentives. This can take the form of cutting corners or shunning responsibility in other areas to meet indicator targets so that employees don't look inferior in the eyes of management. An example from hospital-based performance measurement illustrates this phenomenon. In the early 1990s, interest in comparing various hospitals on their mortality rates for treating certain cardiovascular conditions such as acute myocardial infarction was considerable. The interpretation was that hospitals with lower mortality rates were of higher quality than hospitals with higher mortality rates. This represented faulty logic. Obviously, mortality is not determined only by hospital-based services and processes, but also by a significant number of patient factors, including the severity of the patient's condition, comorbidities, and sociodemographic variables such as age and gender. Presented with the need to improve hospitals' unadjusted mortality rates, administrators had essentially two options. They could either mobilize staff to create better processes with subsequent improved outcomes, or they could try to improve rates by keeping high-risk patients from entering the hospital in the first place. The latter solution is one that the originators of the program did not intend when they began comparing hospital mortality rates. A measurement system intent on exposing bad apples and based on ill-chosen indicators invites management responses and solutions that may improve the measurement but violate the designer's intent.

In addition, an organization that builds an effective performance measurement system and takes advantage of the strategic opportunities inherent in adopting such a system has the advantage of being able to help employees in the organization realize their contribution to excellent organizational performance. For example, even if excellence is achieved in the clinical, service, and cost-effectiveness arenas, different parts of the organizations will have different clinical excellence goals and targets. Yet, the organization's units are striving to achieve similar goals that are conceptually linked. In this manner, measurement is a powerful, integrating force for health care organizations to use in demonstrating that all parts of the organization are contributing to a common vision and mission. It may directly illustrate for each employee how individual measured contributions add to the overall realization of the organization's aims.

ORGANIZATIONAL STAKEHOLDERS AND EFFECTIVE PERFORMANCE MEASUREMENT

Given this organizational culture to use measurement for performance improvement, different managers have different needs and responsibilities with respect to performance measures, depending on the nature of the measure, the level of aggregation, and the degree of detail. In addition, different managers assume different responsibilities for translating performance data into practice.

The Board

The board provides an important oversight function. It is responsible for ensuring that quality and its measurement are anchored to the organization's vision and mission statements. In addition, board members are responsible for holding the executive office and senior leadership accountable for the organization's ability to execute against identified strategies in identifiable and quantifiable ways. The stronger the board's voice in demanding quantifiable information on the organization's progress, the more likely that an effective performance measurement system will be put in place. At the same time, the board assumes leadership in celebrating the organization's successes when strategies and measurable goals have been realized.

Executive Office/Senior Leadership

The executive office and senior leadership share the responsibility of communicating, sustaining, defending, and modeling the organization's vision and mission and creating the links between the vision and mission and quality and its measurement. Similarly, senior leadership has the responsibility for holding employees in all parts of the organization accountable for their ability to provide quantifiable information on organizational strategies, targets, and goals. Senior leadership must ensure that all the organization's departments can provide quantifiable information on their performance through realistic resource allocation. Senior leadership also assumes an important position in ensuring that many dimensions of value are recognized, measured, and rewarded. This requires that individuals throughout the organization subscribe to the same recognizable measurement dimensions. Senior management is also responsible for identifying gaps between current and desired performance and clarifying management's accountability for making credible attempts to close those gaps. Senior leadership also assumes responsibility for ensuring that gains in closing those gaps are celebrated and that those gaps that are not closed are carefully analyzed.

A number of organizations have chosen to convene special teams of top managers dedicated to monitoring organizational quality efforts through sound measurement systems. Typically, these teams are charged with informing and advising the executive office on the progress of organizational quality initiatives, providing analyses of emerging improvement opportunities, and issuing high level recommendations on organizational quality management issues. Although a number of these top managers might already meet in other forums to discuss other issues, the symbolic value of convening a team to specifically address quality improvement and measurement issues based on sound performance data can be substantial.

Middle Management

Middle management has to ensure that organizational strategies are translated into real practice and improvement on the front line. Personnel and work processes need to be organized so that organizational performance goals and targets can be reached. Middle managers provide the lead in identifying specific improvement opportunities, performance goals and targets, and likely tactics that can help fulfill identified goals. An additional key responsibility is encouraging front-line employees to invest and acquire the necessary knowledge and skills to improve performance. Skillful management and support of front-line employees to reach their full potential is a key responsibility of middle management.

CONCLUSION

Improving an organization clearly does not mean hunting down and driving out employees who have been identified as bad apples. When the organization is focused on value, not cost; when those involved recognize that improvement is an ongoing process; and when the environment is one of trust not fear, then that organization is poised for success.

10

Launching a Quality
Initiative: A Case Study

This chapter illustrates how one health system launched a quality initiative and embarked on the journey toward developing
a quality culture. The case study of Allina Health System offers a view of a simultaneous bottom-up and top-down strategy designed to make quality a way of life within an organization. The case
study illustrates a real-life application of the concepts and theories
described in this book.

ASSESSING ALLINA'S QUALITY HISTORY

Allina was formed in 1995 as the result of a merger between a delivery organization and a health plan. Allina Health System is a
not-for-profit health care system serving people living in Minnesota,
western Wisconsin, and eastern North Dakota and South Dakota.
Allina's integrated health care system of doctors, hospitals, and
health plans provides people with a full continuum of care and care
options, from prevention and wellness services such as health
screenings and immunizations to tertiary inpatient care, outpatient
services, home care, hospice, and long-term care services.

The executive office of Allina is shared by two individuals, the
former president and CEO of HealthSpan, the delivery organization, and the former president and CEO of Medica, the health plan.
They have clearly articulated the priorities of the executive office
and have divided its responsibilities. One executive focuses on the
current operational effectiveness of the organization. Reporting to
him are the operations leaders, who are the heads of the major business units, as well as the leaders of finance, human resources, and
legal services. The other executive focuses on strategy, the future direction, and the capacity-building capabilities of the organization.

Reporting to him are those who lead the staff functions of public policy and communications, strategic development, redesign, clinical services, quality and performance effectiveness, information services, and community investment. They are involved continuously in communication, coordination, and strategy development.

The parts that came together to form Allina shared the attribute of having extensive quality histories. However, they had traveled different paths, held different models, and were at differing levels of maturity in their quality journey. This was both a strength and a limitation because leaders and staff members in each part of the organization believed that their philosophy, approach, and results were superior to those in the other part. The use of differing problem-solving methods, language, and foundational quality theories created barriers in the ability of those in the organization to talk about and learn from their experiences. Groups adhering to differing philosophies included the Baldrige quality criteria camp, the Juran followers, the Deming believers, and the Fifth Discipline disciples. In addition to different ways of looking at and understanding quality, different approaches were expressed in the distinctive cultures of each part of the organization. Although this description is of a large, complex, merged organization made up of smaller, previously independent organizations, a similar phenomenon can be observed between divisions, departments and individuals within other organizations in circumstances in which a strong corporate quality culture has not been developed.

The lack of a system approach to quality made it impossible to assess Allina's impact on the care and the service it provided to members, patients, and communities. It also made it difficult to go to the market and demonstrate value. Data and stories from the various parts could be strung together to talk about the whole, but there were breakdowns in the system that hampered efforts at improvement. As a result, many opportunities for improvement went unrealized.

CREATING A NEW LEADERSHIP POSITION AND QUALITY TEAMS

Convinced that care and service quality would be increasingly important to the purchasers and consumers of health care and propelled by the desire for unsurpassed quality in the new company, the executive office created the position of system vice president for quality. It also created two important groups: the Allina Quality Team and the Quality Committee of the Board.

System Vice President for Quality

The system vice president for quality would report directly to the executive office, giving quality high visibility. The position would also provide the individual who accepted this role with the opportunity to participate in the strategy and operations of the company. The role as initially defined was focused on quality improvement and lacked critical components to connect it to measurement, medical policy, and health and clinical improvement. It was, therefore, separate from the product and core competency of the company. It was also separate from the essential improvement instrument of measurement.

Following an extensive process to gain consensus on the topic of quality among leaders from across the organization, the role of system vice president for quality was expanded so that the individual became the accountable vice president for the Allina Quality Team (AQT).

Allina Quality Team

The AQT was launched in the summer of 1995 following the appointment of the system vice president for quality. It received guidance in its formation from external consultants knowledgeable in the field of quality and familiar with the personal commitment, capacity building, and culture required to bring quality to life within a company. Because the AQT members thought they ought to be very intentional in becoming a team, they started by bringing their personal histories and interests forward. They developed their team norms and established working procedures. These ground rules guided them so that they had a well-developed, aligned, and coordinated approach to working with others in the organization. They also clearly articulated the particular area of focus and expertise they would coordinate with other team members.

Figure 10-1 illustrates the design of the team. The team consisted of three individuals, each with a specific area of focus and expertise: the vice president for *medical policy* and medical care redesign focused on the professional provider and evidence-based clinical practice; the vice president for *performance measurement* and improvement focused on information analysis and application; and the vice president for *quality* focused on the development of leadership, culture, and systems for improvement. The team shared responsibility for strategy, accreditation, regulation, standards planning, compliance, operating procedures, and celebrations of gains made.

FIGURE 10-1.   Allina Quality Team

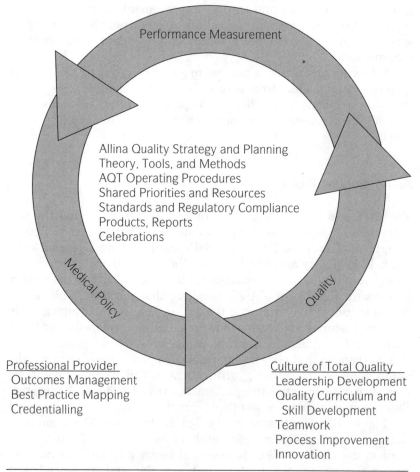

Information Analysis and Application
Key Performance Indicators
Customer Knowledge
Aggregate Clinical Performance
Strategic Quality Planning

Performance Measurement

Allina Quality Strategy and Planning
Theory, Tools, and Methods
AQT Operating Procedures
Shared Priorities and Resources
Standards and Regulatory Compliance
Products, Reports
Celebrations

Medical Policy

Quality

Professional Provider
Outcomes Management
Best Practice Mapping
Credentialling

Culture of Total Quality
Leadership Development
Quality Curriculum and
  Skill Development
Teamwork
Process Improvement
Innovation

Reprinted, with permission, from Allina Heath System, Minnetonka, Minn., 1998.

A quick inventory of the human resources necessary to do the work, once it was defined, yielded a system quality staff that had contributed greatly to the delivery side of the organization throughout its history. A team of internal quality consultants had led the hospitals skillfully through accreditation processes and supported and coached operations and medical staff leaders to meet or exceed compliance standards. They partnered with risk management staff, reporting through the legal services department to conduct audits and risk assessments within the company and complete due diligence procedures before the acquisition of new businesses or medical practices.

Another system resource the team identified was an individual known as a world-class facilitator and trainer in continuous quality improvement methods. This individual was instrumental in working with labor unions and building labor management connections around improvement. Inside the local operating units, quality professionals and resources ranged from a single individual to departments and supporting infrastructures that were appropriately focused on the requirements of their individual operating unit. Some parts of the company had not yet begun to focus on quality and thus lacked individuals with expertise in quality improvement and the infrastructure needed to improve.

Quality Committee of the Board

While the AQT was forming, a quality committee of the board was appointed and chartered. The system vice president for quality was responsible for staffing the committee and preparing them to fulfill their responsibilities for the oversight of quality throughout the organization.

The committee was chaired by a physician board member with a passion for quality and improvement, as evidenced by his practice and governance roles. The committee membership also included a physician who was expert in the field of clinical quality improvement and who served as a resource and mentor for the vice president and the committee. Significant energy was committed to the development of the governance quality structure. A sample board quality committee charter is included in Appendix A at the end of this chapter.

As described in the roles and responsibilities of the board (see Chapter 1), the committee focused its attention on ensuring that quality priorities were established, that appropriate measures were being used, that measures were going back to clinicians on the front line so that they could make improvements, and that results were being reported back to the committee. The committee regularly reviewed quality priorities in detail and reviewed the key measurement indicators of the company's overall performance. Review of the key performance indicators helped determine whether the company and its parts were advancing strategy—was the company executing

FIGURE 10-2.   Sample Agenda of the Quality Committee of the Board

AGENDA

Quality Committee of the Board

- Approval of Minutes
- President's Report
- Work Plan

System Oversight
- Key Performance Indicator Set
  - System Review
  - Business Units
- Patient/Member Experience
  - Survey Results
  - Other
- Clinical Priorities: Measurements and Clinical Integration and Improvements
  - Cardiovascular
  - Diabetes
  - Pregnancy
  - Oncology
  - Asthma
  - Violence
  - Smoking
- Safety
  - Error Reduction
  - Risk
- Ethics

System Integration
- Highlighted Improvements
- Staff Reports
- Discussion

Reprinted, with permission, from Allina Health System, Minnetonka, Minn., 1998.

its strategies according to plan or not? The committee ensured that the operating measures of the company represented a balanced view of performance, not just financial performance. To accomplish this at a glance, the committee challenged the staff to develop a point-in-time data display to view performance along the dimensions of growth, clinical quality, satisfaction and experience, and financial performance. The resulting radar plot display is a display format described in the measurement chapters.

The quality committee of the board also ensured that the organization was complying with regulatory and accreditation standards so that the organization could demonstrate it was a safe place to give and receive care and that improvement was continually taking place. To do this, the committee reviewed the results of all accreditation/regulatory surveys and monitored any corrective actions required. They also reviewed risk and claim experience, processes, follow-up, credentialling processes, and sentinel event analysis. This committee's responsibility was to ensure that management processes were in place to examine findings in a timely manner and prevent failures. Figure 10-2 is an example of an agenda of the quality committee of the board.

Although the committee had delegated responsibility from the board for oversight, the committee had reporting responsibilities back to the board and an obligation to inform and educate the board about improvement and quality performance in the company over time and against external comparisons of best-in-class.

ENGAGING THE COMPANY IN ALLINA'S QUALITY FUNCTION

Concurrent to the early work in developing the governance system, an equally intense effort was made to engage the company in thinking about and influencing the Allina quality function. Over three months, focus groups throughout Allina were held, and groups were invited to respond to the following questions:

- What are your most important successes in the area of quality?
- What do you see as Allina's most important opportunities to improve health care through an integrated quality effort?
- With the formation of the quality team, what is your hope about their ability to add value to the quality initiatives?
- What opportunities or possibilities do you see inside a relationship with the AQT for you?
- To create an integrated approach, what are the most important issues that need to be addressed?
- What would you most like to make sure doesn't get lost in an integrated effort?
- What are you willing to do to partner for success with the quality team?
- What do you see as opportunities for short-term wins in the early stages of the process?

- What advice would you give this team?
- What is the biggest mistake the AQT could make in putting together an Allina quality initiative?
- What do you think are measures to gauge progress?

Most focus groups were conducted by the external consultants. Members of the AQT also conducted "elite interviews" with executive staff members and the operations leaders within the business units. Elite interview refers to the method of interviewing someone who is an expert on the interview topic. It offers open-ended questions, and the interviewer follows the lead of the individual being interviewed. Elite interview does not refer to interviewing an elitist, as some people who were unfamiliar with the field research method inferred initially.

Focus groups went deep into the organization to include frontline employees and providers, as well as managers, quality professionals, union leaders, and positional leaders. In all, more than 300 individuals provided input into the formation of what would become the Allina quality initiative.

Finally, a draft team would help perform a content analysis of the data from focus groups and interviews, and a design team would organize, display, and use the results as the "customer voice" in the quality initiative's design. The next step was to use the findings to inform others throughout the organization about the development of Allina's approach to quality. The work of these two teams is described in the following sections.

Work of the Draft Team

A team was needed to assist the AQT in interpreting the results from the focus groups and interviews and formulating strategy for Allina quality. The team was called the draft team because they would draft the quality strategy for Allina.

The draft team was composed of 10 representative leaders from across Allina. They included the CEO of Allina, a hospital president, the president of diversified services, the president of the health plan, the chairman of the quality committee of the board, a hospital nurse executive, the vice president of strategy and marketing, the vice president of human resources, the vice president of organizational development, and the members of the AQT (the system vice president for quality, the vice president of medical policy and clinical redesign, and the vice president of measurement and performance improvement). The draft team was asked to commit to two, four-hour meetings, an afternoon on one day and the morning of the following day, with homework and think space in the evening between the meetings.

The work of the draft team was composed of visioning, making explicit the individually held principles of quality, synthesizing individual principles into group-held principles, analyzing data, identifying key issues from the data, developing potential long-range strategies for Allina quality, and exploring the framework and relationships required to implement quality strategies.

Create a Shared Vision   The day began with letting members know why they had been invited to participate on the team. Then, each member was asked to describe a high point and a low point in his or her experience with quality. The storytelling provided a rich basis for dialogue on the topic of quality. The stories and subsequent dialogue brought about a realization that quality is very personal, being understood and experienced in different ways by the team members who had assembled.

Figure 10-3 illustrates the scope of beliefs identified by individual draft team members as being essential to quality.

Identify Quality Principles   Next, the draft team members were asked to form two groups to identify from the individual lists the four to six principles of quality that held the most meaning for them as a group. The results of the two groups are displayed in figure 10-4. The results of these two exercises formed the basis for the development of the Allina Quality Principles, listed next, and the Quality Model. Both of these work products became components of the document called the Allina Quality Blueprint. The Blueprint is abstracted and included as Appendix B to this chapter.

The following quality principles were distilled from the draft team's work for Allina:

- The ultimate aim is health improvement.
- Our customers are part of the Allina "system," not just an input.
- The quality journey is inclusive.
- Quality is a discipline.
- Change is constant.

Confirm a Shared Vision   The next agenda item for the first afternoon was a visioning exercise that resulted in the creation of a picture of Allina as a company with unsurpassed quality. The team was given the instruction to create an ennobling, compelling picture of Allina when it had achieved its vision of improving community health improvement.

FIGURE 10-3. Draft Team Members' Responses Listing the Four to Six Principles Believed to Be Essential to Quality

Responder #1
- Improvement of process, results
- Ability to measure
- Decision making supported by objective data
- Customer knowledge
- Customer focus
- Engagement of employees throughout organization

Responder #2
- Customer-driven
- Requirements "delighters"
- Judgments
- Data-supported decision making (strategic and tactical)
- Cycles of evaluation and creativity
- Incremental improvement
- "Breakthrough" innovations
- Development of *capacity* of "human capital" of organization

Responder #3
- Customer knowledge and focus
- Work process management and measurement

- People management and development
- Strategic analysis and planning
- Leadership

Responder #4
- Quality is a value and a discipline that will be integrated into all aspects of work life.
- Quality cannot be managed; it can only be supported/encouraged/mentored/learned.
- Quality can be experienced as well as measured.
- Quality is the integrating principle between people.

Responder #5
- Quality unifies (customers and their requirements/needs).
- Quality simplifies (the work).
- Quality emancipates (through shared goals, ownership as opposed to controls).

The vision was created using a "history of the future" method. What this method does is ask people to imagine themselves in the future and describe what things are like. In this case, what would Allina be like? The team was asked to write a news release about Allina that would appear in the media in February 2001. Figure 10-5 was the product of the visioning exercise.

Given the vision of the future state of Allina at a time when quality would be a way of life, the team was asked next to consider three questions:

FIGURE 10-3. (Continued)

Responder #6
- Focus on clarity about customer requirements
- Continuous improvement of *core* work processes
- Measurement and feedback on *what* matters
- Management accountable for supporting development of processes and systems that support customer requirements
- Everyone as problem solvers

Responder #7
- Quality is a philosophy, a set of principles, a process (as opposed to a structure or form) that supports the achievement and improvement of the services we offer and ennobles those who serve.
- Leadership's demonstration of principles in daily work is essential to achieve quality vision; constancy of purpose.
- Quality work requires trust, a belief in the power and spirit

released when the principles are acted on consistently.
- Quality requires enhanced relationship skills.

Responder #8
- Use data to extent possible for decisions on changes, improvements. Use run control chart whenever measuring a stable process.
- Drive out fear to extent possible.
- To extent possible, utilize process experts and those closest to process to make change.
- Absolute honesty and integrity in process. Avoid generic language to extent possible.
- Encourage mind set that everything that can be measured should be improved continuously.
- Employ quality principles, techniques throughout all key processes of company (including planning, and so on).

Reprinted, with permission, from Allina Health System, Minnetonka, Minn., 1998.

1. What are the things we're doing now that will grow?
2. What are the things we're not doing now, but will be doing?
3. What are the things we will stop doing or will go away?

This exercise was formulated to focus on action that might be required as a result of the vision. It was designed to move teams from concept-developers to action-takers. It also set the stage for the work product to move beyond a consensus statement on paper to real-world strategies that could create positive change. The results

FIGURE 10-4.   Results of Draft Team Quality Principles

Group 1 Results
We will make a positive difference in people's lives.
   How: By creating a quality work environment
   By using: Science and the discipline to practice constantly
              Value of relationship: integrity, trust, respect

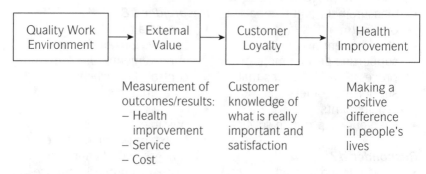

| Quality Work Environment | → | External Value | → | Customer Loyalty | → | Health Improvement |

		Measurement of outcomes/results:	Customer knowledge of		Making a positive
		– Health improvement	what is really important and		difference in people's
		– Service	satisfaction		lives
		– Cost			

Group 2 Results
Quality is:

- How we do everything that we do and an integral aspect of our emerging collaborative management model.
- Driven by our understanding of customers' current and future requirements and needs.
- A discipline, rooted in skills and behaviors.
- Values-based, requiring trust, honesty, integrity, inquiry, and constancy, as well as an orientation balancing short- and long-term perspectives.
- Inclusive, catalyzed by senior leaders, with all management and staff engaged and accountable for contributing.
- Supported by measurement, with results used for strategic and operational decision making.
- Reflected by unending work process improvement and innovations . . . thereby enabling us to better add value to Allina's customers.

of the team's consideration of these three action questions appear in figure 10-6.

Review the Data   The final agenda item for the first afternoon was to review the data from focus groups and interviews. Before the meeting, these results were mailed to the team so that they could prepare for the work they would be asked to do. The team was asked to identify the key strategic forces/issues from the data (figure 10-7).

FIGURE 10-5. Visioning Exercise Results

News Release
Date: February 12, 2001
Allina—Setting the Standard for Quality for the 21st Century

As health care enters a new century, the organization leading the way is Allina, the nation's preeminent integrated health care system.
Allina's history of setting the standard as a quality-driven organization with unmatched clinical excellence is maintained through clarity of vision, a discipline of continuous improvement, excellence in customer service, and investment in employee development.
Throughout the organization, employees have the systems, support, and skills to match their desire to better serve the customer. They are supported in their efforts to innovate. They demonstrate speed of action, and show a remarkable resilience in managing change. Working in teams, employees have come to more fully appreciate and learn from the talents and contributions of their colleagues. Evidence of improvement and innovation is commonplace. Employees are routinely recognized for their contributions and performance.
Customer knowledge and excellence in customer service is a passion for Allina. Allina is designed around the customers; their needs and expectations drive every decision, program, and service. Customers are brought into the organization through a variety of methods so that Allina leaders and employees know their needs, perceptions, preferences, and dreams for health products and services.
Interpersonal relationships are the foundation for the work of Allina, and the source of much of the value and inspiration employees find in their work. These relationships extend into the community, involving Allina's customers and other stakeholders. Employees have a spirit of volunteerism and a connectedness to the communities the organization serves, reflecting Allina's mission of health improvement.
Individuals in leadership positions within Allina have an extraordinarily clear sense of purpose and responsibility. By their leadership, they embody the organization's quality principles. These leadership qualities are shared throughout the organization, evident in individuals with positional leadership responsibilities and individuals who exercise personal leadership based on their talents and contributions.
Allina's systems are designed not only to serve the needs of today, but to adapt quickly to anticipate the work of the future. The organization's technology, processes, and support systems were designed with simplicity, rationality, and responsiveness in mind. In particular, Allina's information systems have been recognized across the country as being accessible, supportive, and flexible—and a major factor in enhancing the customer relationship. For example, an electronic record of an individual's health profile is immediately available to them wherever and whenever they access services.

(Continued on next page)

FIGURE 10-5. (Continued)

Clarity is a major factor in this organization's success. Clarity is supported by specific, measurable goals. By having clear objectives from the start of each project, employees of Allina have been able to eliminate fragmentation and improve clinical and business outcomes. This approach has worked so well for Allina, in fact, that the routine measurements of strategic progress and organizational performance exceed standards set by the National Committee for Quality Assurance, the Joint Commission on Accreditation of Healthcare Organizations, and the Baldrige criteria.

For all their hard work, the staff at Allina have been rewarded with unparalleled customer and employee loyalty, and long-term financial success. Their work has made a positive difference in the lives of the people and the communities they serve.

Allina has done more than set a new standard for health care quality. It is an example of a world-class organization that has thoroughly embedded the principles of quality. Through deliberate, focused efforts and the unyielding commitment of its leaders, Allina has set the standard that others must follow.

FIGURE 10-6. The Future State of Allina When Quality Is a Way of Life

Things We're Doing Now That Will Grow
Work in teams.
Share leadership.
Recognize quality performance.
Grow our relationships with key individuals and groups.
Grow our capacity, capability, character, and courage as individuals and as an organization.
Use measurement for decision making routinely.
Expand our definition of marketplace.
Develop widespread skill in using measurement tools where meaningful and useful.
Increase our value-added work; eliminate non-value added work.
Improve our speed and accuracy.
Increase our playfulness, humor, and sense of enjoyment of one another at work.
Increase our capacity for risk taking and innovation.
Improve our social consciousness and connectedness to our communities.
Grow our healthy community initiative.
Increase our sense of volunteerism.
Expand our redesign efforts so that they become a routine part of what we do.

FIGURE 10-6. (Continued)

Increase heartiness for change.

Increase interest in our commitment to complementary therapies.

Become more sophisticated in how we gather, pool, and retrieve customer feedback.

Increase the number and types of learning opportunities for employees.

Expand our conference center to fill two floors.

Have the Quality Team evolve into R&D.

Increase our internal capacity for people to assume new and creative roles.

Things We're NOT Doing Now But Will Be Doing

Focus on quality outcomes, rather than having them be an afterthought; with the assumption that this supports realizing business outcomes.

Develop a procedure to systematically assess how we are doing related to quality management will be created.

Ensure that all staff functions embrace quality and that the principles of quality are apparent in their processes and relationships.

Create linkages that help us accelerate each other's learning.

Have a cable television service that provides interactive health care information.

Offer individuals and communities health care counselors whom they can access through interactive I.S. or in person to work with them around their choices.

Reduce paper consumption by 75%.

Clarify our purpose, role, responsibility, priority, and values.

Have an empowered front-line employee manage every complaint, and ensure that systems work.

Ensure accuracy of paychecks.

Issue every manager a credit card for all supply purchases, thereby eliminating paperwork and approvals.

Use a smart card for everything.

Provide ways for employees to connect with colleagues across the system to explore questions so that they can learn from each other.

Structurally integrate across Allina with our core processes.

Put an information system that provides accessible data in place.

Create an atmosphere in which employees can walk around with heads held high, making eye contact, taking pride in their work, and actively engaging each other about meaningful work.

Become the Disney of health care.

Cultivate long-term contractual relationships with providers, purchasers, and suppliers.

Become the employer of choice.

Become the health care resource of choice.

(Continued on next page)

FIGURE 10-6. (Continued)

Integrate in such a way that we will not have to prepare for the Joint Commission or Baldrige...we will be there.

Ensure that all employees demonstrate principles and use of tools daily so that there will be examples of regular improvement and innovation.

Ensure that leaders embody principles of quality in how they lead.

Things We Will Change or Eliminate
Eliminate barriers to clinical collaboration: poor relationships, disincentives to collaboration, lack of technology, bad or extraneous measurements.

Eliminate the "mystery" around quality.

Eliminate ignorance about the cost of poor quality.

For patients: Eliminate any aggravation associated with using us.

Replace the erratic billing system.

Eliminate the "us versus them" mentality among internal groups as well as between physicians and Allina.

Stop physicians from using the hospital as a workshop.

Eliminate conflicting incentives.

Cut administrative costs by 50%.

Replace reactive quality initiatives.

Change the traditional structure of medical staffs and departments.

Eliminate fragmentation of quality/QM/QA.

Eliminate excess capacity.

Dramatically reduce paper use.

Reduce internal costs of "churning" among groups, committees, and task forces, as well as enrollees.

Eliminate most emergency care.

Avoid patient-physician mismatch.

Adapted, with permission, from Allina Health System, Minnetonka, Minn., 1998.

The day concluded with the request that team members reflect on the work of the day, paying particular attention to formulating possible strategies around the issues identified in stakeholder focus groups and interviews.

Formulate Quality Strategies The draft team reconvened in the morning and was asked to formulate broad strategic planks that would form a blueprint for quality. They worked through a process of clarifying common issues from their previous work and multivoting to narrow the field to those strategies with the greatest potential of moving Allina toward its vision.

The field of possible strategies was narrowed from 25 to 15. The team was then asked to vote for those strategies they thought would

FIGURE 10-7. Strategic Forces/Issues from the Data

1. Translation of this to/for physicians
2. Decision of what to require/control vs. allowing individual pace of implementation throughout organization
3. Decision of what measures to require as part of the framework
4. Plan to get top management on board
5. Not another quality bureaucracy
6. Common belief that quality will cost money—negative impact on bottom line
7. Caution not to be too ambitious, but not to shoot too low
8. Balance between developing consensus versus moving forward and not asking everyone
9. High expectations for results
10. High expectations for leadership and broad participation
11. Market telling us to get quality implemented
12. Both hope and cynicism about whether anything will happen
13. Call for clarity and focus versus honoring individual history
14. Enthusiasm/energy to tap
15. No real call for resources that we don't have (for example, statistical)
16. Not a lot of discussion about the work—more form and structure
17. Call for practical approaches—fear that it will just be philosophical
18. Lots of references to clinical focus versus other areas
19. Physicians' belief that the quality team will do something *to* them versus *for* them
20. Some call for it to be beyond physicians only
21. Early systems integration efforts, which have not produced results expected
22. Concern about being able to integrate . . . *and* need for a code word for control
23. Some doubt that management will be able to model the principles
24. "Mystery" about where decisions get made . . . and where they should be made

Adapted, with permission, from Allina Health System, Minnetonka, Minn., 1998.

be key for the next three years, using nominal group process. Six high-level strategic planks were proposed by the team to support Allina's long-term evolution as a quality-driven organization. The following strategic planks were identified:

- Transform Allina's planning processes to support quality goals and ensure that they reflect and reinforce quality principles.

- Establish the organizational infrastructure, including technical and facilitative resources, educational vehicles, and communication channels, to support Allina's evolution.
- Advance the systematic and rigorous measurement of Allina's internal and external environments, its efforts, and its impact.
- Enhance Allina's capacity to gather, refine, and disseminate "customer knowledge" as the basis for decision making and action.
- Cultivate shared leadership throughout Allina (for example, boards, senior management, employees, affiliated providers) to ensure its commitment to quality principles.
- Engage physicians, actively and meaningfully, in Allina's commitment to excellence based on quality principles.

The strategic planks were also designed to ensure advancement and create alignment of effort across the company.

The draft team completed its draft of Allina's quality principles and key strategies, with the next steps clearly identified regarding what would happen with their work.

Work of the Design Team

There is only one opportunity to launch something, so it needs to be effective. With this in mind, a design team of 15 members was assembled. The team was so named because their work would be to design a process to bring the work of the draft team to the larger Allina community for endorsement and action. The team was composed of educators, organizational quality professionals, a development consultant, and key stakeholders who understood how to disseminate information and knew the culture of Allina. They were asked to design a launch event that would engage the Allina community, inspire interest in quality, set an expectation for a systems approach, and confirm the draft team's work in formulating the six strategic planks for quality. They began design work before the draft team had finished their work.

Design team members decided that the launch event should:

- Be fun and energizing;
- Have conceptual and applied content;
- Have executive participation, but not be executive dominated;
- Use multiple teaching methods;

- Do something unconventional, so that quality is viewed freshly by participants; and
- Model the principles of quality in the event itself.

The design team planned a large conference that would bring together for the first time executive and operations leaders, physician leaders, quality professionals, and labor leaders. Recognizing diverse ways of receiving and processing information that would be represented in the group assembled, the agenda reflected visual, kinesthetic, and auditory presentation of material. The agenda was also planned to include both high-level conceptual and practical, tactical approaches to the topic.

The design team contracted with the Playback Theater, a group skilled in picking up the unspoken messages communicated by a group. Theater members "played back" in dramatizations to the group the content they interpreted. For example, one group told about the difficulty of letting go of decision making to the front-line manager and their discomfort in trusting that the workforce would respond. The scene the actors dramatized and played back was about loss of control, concerns about interdependence, and the ultimate fear all will turn to chaos without direct management direction. This humorous and poignant drama opened a new level of conversation and insight about the implications of a quality journey in workforce empowerment.

This playback technique was used throughout the conference to move discussion from superficial to substantive issues, as well as to teach and entertain. The one-day conference, titled "Shaping the Future of Quality at Allina," was divided into two parts. The morning was designed to develop community, explore messages in the compressed data of stakeholder input, and confirm the work of the draft team. The afternoon was designed to allow participants to form a work group around the strategy that held the most interest for them. Letting people form their own groups based on their interest instead of assigning groups resulted in people selecting one of the six strategies to develop specific tactics to implement.

The product of the conference was the Allina Blueprint for Quality. A conference agenda is shown in figure 10-8. Prework sent to all participants included the following information and a request to prepare for the conference:

- Results of focus groups, surveys, and interviews about Allina quality: The raw data is available to you.
- Prework for the day prepared by an expert draft team: This section contains an introduction of the draft team and the

FIGURE 10-8.   Agenda for Quality Conference

AGENDA FOR QUALITY CONFERENCE
- Welcome and context
- Drop your title at the door
- Group demographics—movement/travel

  - Area of practice
  - Geographic location of practice
  - Optimism about quality at Allina

- Data Analysis: Implications
- 3 Quality Stories and Playback

  - Executive
  - Front-line provider
  - Quality team

- Work of Draft Team

  - Principles
  - Strategies

- Confirmation
- Lunch
- Open-Space Tactics Development
- Wrap-Up and Next Steps

Reprinted, with permission, from Allina Health System, Minnetonka, Minn., 1998.

process used to produce the products that will serve as the basis for our work together. The products include the following:

- Visions of the future state of Allina when quality is a way of life
- Principles of quality held high by each draft team participant, as synthesized by the two team subgroups, in response to the task: "From the generated list, what are the key principles you agree upon to guide quality for Allina?"
- The draft team's identification of strategic issues emerging from the data
- Identification of possible strategies in response to the issues
- The six long-range strategies to provide direction to Allina quality
- The model of the Allina Quality Team and the operating principles

The AQT synthesized the work of the conference into a single document. The document, or Blueprint, was presented to the quality committee of the board, executive office, senior management, the labor management committee of Allina, and the business unit operations groups. This grassroots document was endorsed by the executive office and board as the quality plan for the health system. Because of the process used to create the plan, it had ownership throughout the company before its implementation.

The Blueprint, provided as an addendum to this chapter, is a synthesis of quality planning for Allina and is broadly owned by all operational leaders across Allina who incorporate it into their planning and operations.

MANAGING IMPLEMENTATION OF THE QUALITY BLUEPRINT

A group was formalized to manage the rollout and implementation of the Blueprint for Quality. Quality professionals from all operating areas across Allina came together to become the Allina Quality Network, facilitated by the system vice president for quality. Two elements the network identified as essential to support the implementation of the Blueprint were a video that provided the context for the Blueprint and a manager's user's manual. The video shows real stories and commentary about Allina quality from the executive office through all levels, functions, and services of the company, including consumers. The second element, a manager's user's manual, offers a guide for managers to use with their staff to bring the Blueprint for Quality to life. The video, Blueprint, and user's manual are tools provided to all current managers and to new managers at orientation. The video is used in employee orientation and at functions throughout the company. It is also provided to community, consumer and purchaser groups to illustrate, from the voices and experiences of Allina consumers and employees, the company commitment to quality.

CONCLUSION

The design of a quality initiative requires both executive and grassroots involvement to create ownership within the company. Engagement of the company needs to be an intentional strategy and viewed as an investment in creating change. Key steps described in this case study included: executive and leadership commitment, customer voice, a draft team, a stakeholder conference, a Blueprint for action, and a dissemination strategy.

Sample Board Quality Committee Charter

ROLES AND RESPONSIBILITIES/GUIDELINES/RULES

I. Roles and Responsibilities

The Quality Committee has two broad roles and sets of responsibilities. The first is to directly oversee, on behalf of the board of directors, quality assurance and improvement processes for the system. The second is to enhance quality across and throughout the system. The latter encompasses aspects of key process and clinical integration and the service experience of members and patients within the system.

In fulfilling these responsibilities, the Committee expressly relies on the confidential protections afforded by law to review activities conducted for the purpose of reducing morbidity and mortality and improving the care and services provided to patients and members.

A. System Oversight

As the governing body, the board of directors is charged by law and by the Joint Commission on Accreditation of Healthcare Organizations (Joint Commission) and National Committee on Quality Assurance (NCQA) with ensuring the quality of care rendered by the system through its various divisions. To meet this responsibility, the board of directors has formed a Quality Committee, whose responsibilities include the following:

1. Reviewing, monitoring, and approving system quality assurance, improvement, and resource utilization plans

2. Overseeing and approving medical staff and health plan credentialling processes

      3. Initiating inquiries, studies, and investigations within the scope of duties delegated to the Committee

      4. Performing, on behalf of the board of directors, such other activities as are required by the Joint Commission, NCQA, and other regulatory bodies

      5. Performing such other activities as requested by the board of directors

      6. Submitting reports and recommendations to the board of directors on its activities

  B. System-Wide Integration

      1. To enhance the quality of service and care provided throughout the system and to encourage a consistent standard of care, the Quality Committee may monitor the quality assurance and improvement activities of system business units by requesting reports.

      2. The Quality Committee may initiate inquiries and make suggestions for improvement.

      3. The Quality Committee will conduct ongoing reviews of the following key areas:

        a. Customer experience

        b. Community health improvement

        c. Clinical outcomes

        d. Safety

        e. Workforce quality

        f. Accreditation and regulatory review

        g. Ethics framework

      4. To further enhance the quality integration of the system, the Quality Committee shall monitor the progress of the quality improvement process and serve as a champion of issues concerning quality to the board of directors and its other committees.

  C. Reports

  The Quality Committee shall make regular reports to the board of directors on its activities and findings.

II. Guidelines

Committee guidelines are designed to govern the operations of the Committee.

  A. Handling of Confidential Documents

  Confidential documents will be distributed in advance of meetings with the standard agenda package. They will be separately identified, numbered, and logged. They will be collected after review at meetings. A return envelope will be forwarded to Committee members unexpectedly unable to attend a meeting so that they will have a convenient method of returning these materials.

    B. Standard Agenda

        The standard agenda for the Committee shall include the following:

        1. President's report

        2. Key performance indicator set—system

        3. Key performance indicator set—business units

        4. Clinical and health improvement priorities

        5. Ethics

        6. Safety: risk management

        7. Highlighted improvements

        8. Staff reports

        Reports may not be made on each agenda item in each meeting.

III. Rules

    Authority to act for board of directors:

    Composition:

    Recommended size:

    Quorum requirement:

    Meeting schedule:

    Staff support:

    Guests:

Blueprint for Quality *

CONTENTS

BLUEPRINT PURPOSE

The Allina Blueprint is written to outline the fundamental responsibility for quality of the governing board members, physician leaders, senior executives, quality management professionals, managers, and employees that comprise Allina.

---

*Reprinted, with permission, from *Blueprint for Quality,* Allina Health System, Minnetonka, Minn., 1995.

The Blueprint outlines the long-term investment and strategies for us as we extend and deepen quality improvement as part of the culture of Allina Health System. This is a living document to be modified and enhanced as our knowledge expands and our experience requires. The Blueprint focus is in two areas: building a culture or context in which learning, improvement, experimentation, and innovation flourish, *and* providing focus, clarity, and relevance to support front-line workers in meeting the needs of our customer.

The Allina Blueprint for Quality was produced from stakeholder requirements and participation in its design.

Specific initiatives—for example, prioritized clinical areas of focus for Allina, prioritized community health improvement areas, and key processes for improvement across Allina—are identified by groups designated to do so from across Allina through the Allina senior management. These provide clarity of focus for quality improvement initiatives.

INTRODUCTION

This blueprint is a product of the initial engagement strategy in which stakeholders from the Allina community came together to create a shared vision and six strategic planks to actualize the vision for quality. This shared vision for quality will serve as a vehicle to achieve Allina's overall vision.

Allina's vision is to be the recognized innovator in community health improvement. This vision recognizes that the world we live in is changing in significant ways. Our society is aging. Homicide and suicide are now greater threats than illness in many communities. New antibiotic-resistant diseases are on the rise. Divorce, stress, and a changing work environment are causing numerous mental health and family problems.

Given these changes, Allina realizes that it is not enough to provide quality health care to those who are ill or injured. We must find the root cause of health problems-whether it be violence, smoking, or stress-and find ways to intervene before people end up in our emergency rooms, clinics, and hospitals. But we will not make this journey alone. Working with other corporations, agencies, and community organizations, Allina will find innovative ways to improve the health of all the communities we serve.

Fundamentally, everything Allina does helps us reach this vision. From wellness programs at employer sites to farm safety programs in rural communities, we are constantly looking for better ways to improve community health.

Key assumptions underlying the development of the blueprint are as follows:

- The ultimate aim is health improvement.
- Customers are part of the Allina "system," not just an input.
- Our quality journey is inclusive.
- Quality is a discipline.
- Change is constant.

The engagement strategy was an intentional design to enroll the Allina community in the quality journey and create the environment for inclusive participation and ownership in the design of the Quality Blueprint.

Hundreds of stakeholders were involved in the process from the front line directly caring for and serving customers, business unit managers, leaders, executives, and board members.

DEFINITION OF QUALITY

Quality at Allina is a value and a discipline of knowledge, skills, and practices to achieve excellence in products, services, and environment based on the requirements, perceptions, and future needs of our customer. *Quality is how we work in Allina.* The focus is defect or error reduction, reduction of waste, and innovation to meet new and emerging customer needs.

ALLINA QUALITY PRINCIPLES

A set of principles characterizes any quality-driven organization. They apply to all operations and staff functions, and all individuals. In combination, they guide an approach for employees to use in their individual work, in their work with each other, and in relationships with Allina's customers and other key stakeholders.

Allina's quality principles include the following:

- Leadership
- Customer-focus
- Results-focus
- Shared meaning and values
- Learning through cycles of inquiry and evaluation
- Statistical thinking

- Data-based decision making
- A systems or process flow perspective
- Continual improvement

FRAMEWORK

The framework adapted for Allina to pursue organizational excellence is the Malcolm Baldrige criteria. *The framework ties all the major functions together and creates the alignment necessary* to experience the definition of quality and apply the principles as we go about our work in service to the customer. It is the supportive structure that weaves the quality principles throughout the organization. Baldrige was identified as the broad organizing framework because it:

- Emerged from the Allina community.
- Provides best-of-practice capability.
- Is nonprescriptive.
- Emphasizes alignment and deployment.
- Applies to organizations including health care.

A model for the framework, which is adapted as the Allina framework, is displayed below:

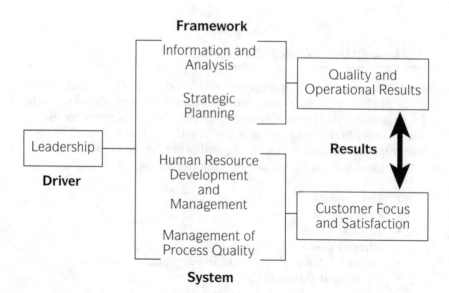

ROLES AND RESPONSIBILITIES

The Employees

The work of quality is everyone's responsibility in Allina. It is a value, a pursuit of curiosity, a relentless pursuit of learning, of eliminating waste and of improvement. The principles of quality are embodied by all members of the Allina community. We are all leaders and followers in the quality journey.

All employees have in their role the following:

- Assume responsibility for improvement and the elimination of error and waste.
- Live the quality principles.
- Serve the purpose of the organization.
- Challenge contradictions to values and principles.
- Participate in change.

Leadership

The Board   The board is ultimately responsible for the work Allina does and the quality of that work. Responsibilities include the following:

- Ensuring that improvement is occurring
- Requiring constancy of purpose in the quality journey
- Holding senior leadership accountable for results
- Ensuring community needs are met
- Leading celebrations of gains made
- Improving its own methods

Senior Leadership   The role of senior leadership is to set strategic direction, focus the quality imperatives and ensure the operations of the company. Obligations and responsibilities include the following:

- Creating, sustaining, and perpetuating shared vision
- Keeping the customers and their experiences at the center of our work
- Monitoring measured performance and naming the gaps that must be closed between actual and targeted results
- Nurturing commitment to quality principles and leading by example
- Insisting on improving the rate of change to achieve best-in-class results

- Providing resources for knowledge and skill development in innovation and learning
- Establishing accountability for trust and improvement
- Recognizing gains made
- Holding people accountable for changes that must take place at the front line

Managers

Managers nurture the environment and develop the staff resources to integrate the quality principles into the workplace. They also model quality principles. Responsibilities include the following:

- Anchoring the work to the vision and mission of Allina
- Planning for quality improvement
- Creating an environment of trust and accountability for improvement
- Intelligently creating and managing change
- Providing development opportunities for staff
- Encouraging participation by staff
- Modeling the way

Quality Resources and Network Members

The Quality Team and the Quality Network* members have the responsibility to accelerate improvement, catalyze innovation, and design the infrastructure for improvement and learning. Responsibilities include the following:

- Catalyzing the incorporation of quality principles throughout and across Allina
- Creating infrastructure and alignments for organizational learning and improvement
- Promoting opportunities for improvement and innovation
- Providing expert consultation and technical assistance within the Allina community
- Importing new ideas, knowledge, and technologies
- Deploying knowledge, skills, and practices throughout Allina
- Enabling the process of change
- Embodying quality principles

---

*Quality Network members are those individuals throughout Allina who have responsibility by job title, for coordinating local quality efforts.

Allina Employees*
Understand quality principles and the key areas of organizational performance, and incorporate these concepts into daily work

Managers
Manage the environment, develop the staff resources and skills to integrate the quality principles into the workplace, and model quality principles

Leaders
Cultivate the environment, guide the incorporation of quality principles throughout Allina, and lead by example

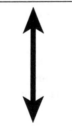
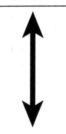

Key areas of organizational performance as defined by:

- Mission/vision
- Learning and innovation
- Consumer (patient/member/population) health status
- Customer satisfaction
- Other stakeholder satisfaction
- Administrative and business results, including financial indicators
- Community health and public responsibilities
- Human resource performance/development
- Organizational performance relative to competitors and similar health organizations

Focus on results (outcomes) characterized by:

- Selection/development of techniques, tools, systems
- Focus on common requirements while fostering better understanding, communication, and sharing while supporting creativity in approaches
- Focus on improvement (learning) cycles

*Allina Employees includes employees and volunteers, management, health care staff and contracted providers, board members, suppliers, and community partners.

Reprinted, with permission, from Allina Health System, Minnetonka, Minn., 1998.

Physicians

Allina physicians are in all groups and job responsibilities. They are direct providers of care and work with Allina. Some are employed; some are position leaders, informal leaders, and managers. Some physicians are clinical quality improvement leaders by job description.

QUALITY FUNCTIONS AND ALLINA QUALITY STAFF

Quality Functions

Areas of current work and responsibility within Allina are associated with compliance, safety, quality improvement and include functions required by regulators, accrediting bodies, and liability insurers. Included are the following:

- Regulatory compliance and accreditation
- Practice profiling and peer review
- Credentialling
- Safety/risk management
- Quality control and assurance
  - Drug use and evaluation
  - Adverse drug reactions
  - Blood use
  - Pharmacy and therapeutics
  - Procedure monitoring
  - Medical records
  - Infection control
- Data collection, measurement, and reporting
- Quality improvement initiatives

In these areas, the Allina quality staff and network provide consultation and education as requested and monitor the aggregated experience across Allina to ensure processes are in control, identify improvement opportunities and best-practices, and catalyze learnings.

The Allina quality and performance effectiveness staff activities focus in three areas:

1. Promoting new opportunities through scanning the environment for improvement
2. Building linkages and relationships to create new knowledge

3. Preventing rigidity of thinking through promoting curiosity and a systemic view through rigorous measurement of performance

The Allina quality and performance effectiveness activities with the Allina Quality Council include the following:

- System-wide quality planning, quality control, and quality improvement
- Development and deployment of methods, tools, techniques, and expert resources in change management (for example, improvement, design, re-engineering, innovation)
- Facilitation training, development, and network expertise
- Provision of technical expert resources in measurement and analysis
- Clinical care outcome design and pilot study design
- Board and executive quality leadership development

QUALITY LONG-RANGE STRATEGIC PLANKS

Six strategic planks were identified to support Allina's long-term evolution as a quality-driven organization. The ultimate aim of these strategic planks is to improve the quality of health care; and to improve value for patients, members, and communities by decreasing the burden of illness.

Six long-term strategic planks serve to advance the work of quality:

1. Cultivate shared leadership throughout Allina to steward its commitment to quality principles and establish accountability for improvement (for example, boards, senior management, employees, unions, affiliated providers).
2. Engage physicians, actively and meaningfully, in Allina's commitment to excellence based on quality principles.
3. Transform strategic planning processes to reflect and reinforce quality principles.
4. Enhance Allina's capacity to gather, refine, and disseminate "customer knowledge" as the basis for decision making and action.
5. Establish the organizational infrastructure, including technical and facilitative resources, educational vehicles, and communication channels, to support Allina's evolution.

6. Advance the systematic and rigorous measurement of Allina's internal and external environments, its efforts, and their results.

The following table highlights the relationship between the strategic planks and the Malcolm Baldrige criteria.

Quality Framework/Strategic Plank Relationships

Baldrige Category	Strategic Plank
1.0 Leadership	#1: Cultivate Shared Leadership
	#2: Engage Physicians
2.0 Information and Analysis	#6: Advance Measurement
3.0 Strategic Planning	#3: Transform Strategic Planning
4.0 HR Development and Management	#5: Establish Infrastructure
5.0 Process Management	#5: Establish Infrastructure
6.0 Organizational Performance Results	#6: Advance Measurement
7.0 Customer Knowledge, Relationship, and Satisfaction	#4: Enhance "Customer Knowledge"
	#6: Advance Measurement

LEADERSHIP

1. Cultivate shared leadership throughout Allina to steward its commitment to quality principles and establish accountability for improvement (for example, boards, senior management, employees, unions, affiliated providers). Tactics to achieve this strategy include the following:

   • Design curriculum and forums to foster the development of both positional and emerging leaders to create and lead a quality-driven company.
   • Have Allina leaders complete launch curriculum.
   • Implement coaching strategies to enhance leadership performance, focusing on attributes of leaders.
   • Participate in labor-management strategies.
   • Identify vehicles for demonstrating and symbolizing shared leadership in practice throughout Allina.
   • Provide Board of Trustee orientation and ongoing education in quality responsibilities.

- Partner with human resources on Allina leadership development, strategies, change-management skills, and employee learning and skill-building.

PHYSICIAN ENGAGEMENT

2. Engage physicians, actively and meaningfully, in Allina's commitment to excellence based on quality principles.* Tactics to achieve this strategy include the following:

   - Partner with human resources and clinical services to develop curriculum and training modules addressing core competencies (for example, interpersonal/team skills, systems thinking, problem-solving skills, tools and methods of improvement based on needs assessment, key requirements, data sources).
   - Establish communication linkages (built on I.S. technology).
   - Develop physician champions for quality throughout Allina.
   - Implement pilot projects to improve issues in the practice setting that matter to physicians.
   - Establish a resource package to support physician involvement and interest in improvement efforts.
   - Develop incentives (not necessarily only financial) to support physician participation in training and projects based on what is meaningful to physicians.
   - Coordinate improvement efforts by building on work-in-progress (leveraging and focusing activities to increase efficiency and reduce competing demands for physician time).
   - Engage physicians in the process through meaningful participation avenues (ask physicians about barriers and issues that matter to them and incorporate their perspectives in definition of Allina quality values and principles).
     - The recurring theme from the practice community is for Allina to establish clear, system-wide clinical

---

*Meaningful engagement means the identification of strategies that relate to multiple roles and relationships of physicians in Allina, for example, clinician, patient-advocate, manager, business person in the running of a private practice setting, leader.

priorities that have meaning for the caregivers and their patients in a real practice environment. Necessary components are including the cost of care and cost of poor quality in the definitions of quality and integrating these concerns into the quality process.

– A strategic priority is supporting and sustaining the development of physician champions and clinical mentors across the system; and resources to promote this strategy must include communication.

– Physician leaders can be a driving force for quality in the organization if leadership is defined, if physicians can be engaged (front-line caregivers), and if physicians are included in ways that support the values and training that physicians bring to the process. These include an understanding that:

–Traditional care is individual patient-focused, not population-focused.

–Physician personalities and styles may be in perceived conflict with quality principles—autonomy, personal, not team accountability.

–Creativity and innovation are necessary values, as well as focus on reducing unintended variations in practice.

–Legal liabilities are real issues.

–Traditional physician learning is an "apprenticeship" model—individually oriented.

Allina clinical care strategy involves multidisciplinary and interdisciplinary best-of-practice definitions using clinical experts from all disciplines to define key requirements for care and health improvement strategies. Clinical priorities are as follows:

- Colorectal cancer
- Breast cancer
- Pediatric asthma
- Pregnancy care
- Diabetes care
- Cardiovascular care
- Community priorities are violence/intentional injury and smoking

The Allina Quality Council evaluates opportunities, sets clinical priorities, and establishes implementation strategies across the system. This group includes physician and nurse leadership.

STRATEGIC PLANNING

3. Transform strategic planning processes to reflect and reinforce quality principles.
   Tactics to achieve this strategy include the following:

   - Identify quality goals and integrate in the planning process.
   - Integrate quality, program, financial, and strategic needs in the planning cycle.
   - USE the Malcolm Baldrige framework to integrate all dimensions of planning related to business results.
   - Continue orientation of planning cycle toward accommodation of a long view.
   - Introduce Hoshin-Kanri goal planning to create alignment of effort (description displayed in Appendix I) (Reference: Melum, Mara Minerva, *Breakthrough Leadership: Achieving Organizational Alignment through Hoshin Planning*, Chicago: American Hospital Publishing, 1995).

Allina will continue its efforts to design a planning process that ensures the following general content areas are explicitly addressed:

- Customer knowledge
- Competitive quality performance
- Product and service performance
- Reduction in deficiencies
- Improvement of macro processes
- Costs of poor quality

The process of planning contains the following attributes:

- Physician involvement
- Stakeholder involvement
- Development that is interactive and engaging
- Driven by customer requirements
- Drives financial/resource requirements
- Systemic perspective
- Cycle of evaluation for planning
- Prioritized and focused
- Highly communicated
- Descriptive of milestones

CUSTOMER PERSPECTIVE

4. Enhance Allina's capacity to gather, refine, and disseminate "customer knowledge," the basis for decision making and action at the front line of care and service.
    Tactics to achieve this strategy include the following:

    - Link customer knowledge to strategic planning and action plan development.
    - Increase information sharing and coordination of efforts (establish customer group advisory bodies for the following: employees, physicians, patients, members, employer purchasers).
    - Incorporate customer requirements in surveys with coordination of survey administration and trending of results.
    - Enhance customer knowledge database (build on market research library capabilities).
    - Experiment with point-of-service vehicles for incorporating customer knowledge.
    - Develop training modules (customer knowledge template, collection processes, interpretation, application of results) for management, staff, and physicians, and address listening skills and capacity of front line staff and caregivers to act.
    - Increase employee customer contact time (even those not typically in contact roles).
    - Engage I.S. support (technical assistance in developing customer knowledge "brain").
    - Collaborate with HR in revision of job descriptions relative to acquisition and use of customer knowledge.
    - Involve customers in redesign efforts in five areas of clinical priority.
    - Partner with marketing and planning to bring quality expertise to interpretation and use of customer data.
    - Profound understanding of our "customer" is the anchor for integrated strategic planning. Like the Measurement Strategic Plank, results of the Key Customer Requirement and Customer Satisfaction Survey Strategy projects provide the foundation for this work. Building on the emerging market research library, increased sharing of customer requirement information will be supported and increasingly anticipated by Allina senior management.
    - The Picker survey instrument is a key tool for understanding customer experience of care and services and focusing improvements.

INFRASTRUCTURE

5. Establish the organizational infrastructure, including technical and facilitative resources, educational vehicles, and communication channels, to support Allina's the front line. Tactics to achieve this strategy include the following:

- Establish Quality Resource Directory, a catalog of improvement initiatives, key learnings, and contact people from across Allina.
- Operate Allina Quality Network (technical, implementation oriented).
- Operate Allina management Quality Council (strategic focus).
- Provide Change Management Tool Kit.
- Provide facilitation support and training.
- Implement systematic performance measurement system.
- Develop measurement panels for clinical priorities with the Clinical Action Groups, support improvement initiatives and pilot studies.
- Improve regulatory and compliance process.
- Sponsor education and training experience: measurement, improvement, systems thinking.
- The following resources are available:
  - *Change Management Tool Kit:* Allina methods and tools for quality improvement and redesign/re-engineering were identified, including definitions, problem-solving tools and methods, dissemination, and training in use of the tool kit.
  - *Facilitation:* Curriculum, training, design, and sustainment of a facilitator practice network for Allina has been developed and implemented.
  - *Performance Measurement:* Science and tools, training in question formulation, measurement, analysis, and conversion of information to action.
  - *Patient/Member Experience:* Customer requirements are documented; customer perspective is systematically obtained, analyzed, and communicated. Processes to provide best-in-class service quality are developed.
  - *Clinical Action Groups (CAGs):* Cross-functional clinical care management teams representing system-wide responsibility, have been charged with implementing the best-of-practice (BOP) models for a

particular disease/population group. This integration management group consists of caregivers, stakeholders, and customers, and will include representation from I.S., health plans, quality, patient care, medical policy, health improvement, and finance. This group will identify key priorities and strategies for effectively implementing the BOP design.

Policy

The quality strategy also requires the review of organizational policy to ensure congruence and support of Allina's quality principles.

1. Manager and employee evaluation based on contribution to quality
2. Rewards and recognitions for contributions to quality
3. Supplier selection and retention requirements
4. Assessment of competitive quality performance: How do we monitor and react?
5. Products and services development and performance requirements
6. Customer listening and relationship management
7. Employee participation in the quality process: Who participates and under what circumstances/conditions? Will process improvement be mandated as part of all operating plans?
8. Employee apprehension: How will we respond to questions about job security in the context of quality improvement.

MEASUREMENT

6. Advance the systematic and rigorous measurement of Allina's internal and external environments, its efforts, and their results.
   Tactics to achieve this strategy include the following:

   - Use key performance indicator sets for Allina and the principal business units to measure performance and advance strategy.
   - Use performance measurement indicator panels for the five Allina-wide clinical priorities to measure performance and drive improvement.

- Clarify definitions and develop an explicit performance measurement model.
- Partner with I.S. in clarification of data sources, development of tools, design of reporting vehicles, and data repository development.
- Enhance capacity to obtain and apply comparative data (for example, competitive, benchmark, regional/national norms).
- Develop training modules regarding measurement issues (for example, question formulation, data collection, data interpretation, result application for improvement) for business leaders, staff and physicians.
- Enhance external interface (for example, payors, regulators, accreditors) regarding performance measurement.
- Provide consultants and resources.

Description

Efforts to advance this strategic plank build on the foundation of major projects completed in 1995 (Key Customer Requirements, Key Performance Indicators, Customer Satisfaction Survey Strategy). The three Allina-wide projects, pursued in parallel due to the urgency caused by rapid organizational and market change are depicted below:

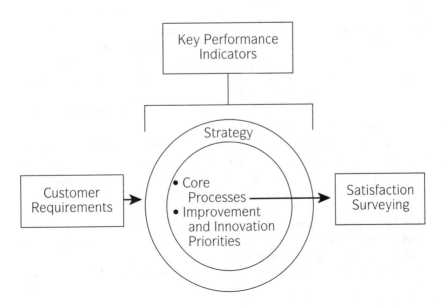

APPENDIX I: QUALITY PLANNING AND DEPLOYMENT

In the function of quality planning, Hoshin-Kanri is an approach to the development and execution of quality strategies to focus the efforts of Allina to achieve breakthroughs of high performance for customers. The Hoshin process is a method to align the organization to achieve results. Hoshin planning and goal setting is also a deployment technique for strategy implementation.

A brief description of the Hoshin process follows:

Hoshin Goals

Main Purpose	Organizational problem solving for breakthroughs
Focus	Business capabilities in meeting/exceeding customer, consumer, and stakeholder expectations and perceptions
Execution	Teams
Responsibility	Participation
Methodology	Quality principles, methods, tools
Time Horizon	Annual activity aligned with long-term goal
Review	Periodic progress on process and results
Objective Priority	Vital few for competitive advantage
Decision Basis	Facts and data
	Customer perspective

APPENDIX II: GLOSSARY OF TERMS

Accreditation: Accreditation is one form of external review. The word technically means to certify or credential, and in the realm of health care, it generally means that a delivery system has met certain established standards that represent a minimally acceptable level of performance. Accreditation of a health care system is considered by many to be a seal of approval on which purchasers and consumers can base decisions.

Algorithm: A format for presenting a clinical practice guideline that consists of a structured flowchart of decision steps and preferred clinical management pathways. An algorithm prescribes what sequence of steps to take given particular circumstances or characteristics (for example, a particular lab result). (Algorithms, or step-by-step approaches to solving problems, were invented by the Persian mathematician, Al-khaforizmi, in the ninth century, as a method for solving arithmetic problems.)
Source: Office of Technology Report & Assessment, U.S. Congress, 1994.

Allina Clinical Action Group: The Clinical Action Group (CAG) is a multidisciplinary, multidimensional action/accountability group made up of key clinical leaders within the Allina Health System. The CAG will adopt Allina's three strategic goals: (1) maintain consistent standards and process of care; (2) create and promote a culture of collaboration; and (3) implement a method to transition to health improvement. To define the context of care for the community, design and deliver integrated activities which focus on health and a continuum of care. This group will oversee the best-of-practice design teams and be responsible for integrating this work system-wide.

Allina way: A manner and method of doing work and a mode of behaving that is identified with and distinguishes Allina. It is the result of the intentional development of a culture of shared purpose, values, and clarity. It is an expectation that an individual would experience the same service quality throughout Allina, regardless of the point of entry.

Appropriateness: The degree to which the care/intervention provided is relevant to the patient's clinical needs, given the current state of knowledge.

Appropriateness of service: This measures whether a particular service that was provided is actually indicated in the care of a given patient. It also measures whether a needed service has not been provided. Of particular importance are diagnostic procedures, medications, and therapeutic procedures.

Availability: The degree to which the appropriate care/intervention is available to meet the needs of the patient served.

Best-of-practice: The "best-of-practice" exercise is the framework for clinical decision making/decision support tools. The best-of-practice exercise is a process to engage physicians in a clinical forum that develops the tools to integrate clinical information technologies, define key clinical requirements, and build Allina system-wide methodologies to measure clinical outcomes and improve health care.

Best-of-Practice Design Team: Provider partners and clinical champions come together to identify the outcomes for a disease/population group and the key requirements for care that include input from the customer. They determine the costs of poor quality, what the focus of outcomes should be, and long-term strategies for population health. This results in a best-of-practices (BOP) model that includes care paths and guidelines for use by clinicians in order to achieve the goal of uniformity of decision making and uniformity of patient care at a specific setting.

Case management: The methodology that is used to ensure that the highest quality, most efficient care is provided to an individual member patient and/or across a continuum of care, services, and time.

Catalyst: A leader who is enlisting and enthusing; making the case for radical change, creating the sense of urgency, and informing about the potential.

Clinical practice guidelines: These are systematically developed statements to assist practitioner and patient decisions about appropriate health care for specific clinical circumstances.
Source: Institute of Medicine and AHCPR.

Clinical Action Group (CAG): A cross-functional clinical care management team representing system-wide responsibility, charged with implementing the best-of-practices (BOP) models for a particular disease/population group. This integration management group consists of caregivers, stakeholders, and customers, and will include representation from I.S., health plans group, quality, patient care, medical policy, health improvement, and finance. This group will identify key priorities and strategies for effectively implementing the BOP design.

Clinical care model: Allina's clinical care model is one of Allina's critical integration strategies, bringing together public policy, health improvement, care management, quality, delivery services, and outcomes management. It links existing resources to improve the health of members and patients we serve. The clinical care model process creates goals and sets priorities for key disease or patient groups identified as clinically important to integrate from the corporate level. The result of the clinical care model is clinical excellence, and the process and results are measurable over time.

Clinical excellence: The result of applying the clinical care model. It is the tangible outcome of care delivered to every person cared for.

Clinical integration: The corporate commitment to develop and standardize systems to support clinical care.

Clinical quality: Clinical quality has two components: (1) Technical: The skill and competence of people and the systems, procedures and equipment that perform reliably and effectively in a way that is quantifiable. (2) Experiential: The subjective experience of the healing relationship that is developed through the customer's interactions with the caregiver and the environment where care and services are provided.

Community health improvement: An Allina strategy that results in coordinated improvement interventions made at the individual, community, and system (for example, public policy) levels to deal effectively with the causes of poor health.

Context: The culture or work environment that we want and need to create excellence and superior results.

Continuity: The degree to which the care/intervention for the patient is coordinated among practitioners, between organizations, and across time.

Corporate: Shared by all members of a unified group, common, joint.

Source: Webster's New World Dictionary of the American Language, Second College Edition, 1980.

Culture: The ideas, customs, skills, arts, etc., of a given people in a given period. A way of seeing things; a way of making sense.

Source: Webster's New World Dictionary of the American Language, Second College Edition, 1980.

Customers: Parties who receive and/or pay for our services (this includes consumers, employer purchasers, and public-sector purchasers).

Customer-focused: A fundamental property of an organization or individual that reinforces the importance of identifying and meeting customer requirements as *the* basis for long-term success; this property is reflected in major management systems, including planning, process and product design, human resource development, performance review, and customer relationship management.

Effectiveness: The degree to which the care/intervention is provided in the correct manner, given the current state of knowledge, to achieve the desired/projected outcome(s) for the patient. The effectiveness of health care relates to professional and support staffs' ability to perform in a manner that ensures that patients achieve the most desirable outcome. In addition, effectiveness involves minimizing risks to patients, insofar as is possible, and documenting patients' health status and the care provided accurately and completely.

Efficacy: The degree to which the care/intervention used for the patient has been shown to accomplish the desired/projected outcomes.

Efficiency: The ratio of the outcomes (results of care/intervention) for a patient to the resources used to deliver the care.

Evaluation: The review and assessment of the quality and/or appropriateness of an important aspect of care for which a pre-established level of performance (threshold for evaluation) has been reached during monitoring activities.

Front line: Where Allina directly meets the customer in delivering products, care, and services.

Function: Goal-directed, interrelated series of processes, such as quality assessment and improvement functions.

Indicator: A quantitative value that reflects the condition and/or direction over time of performance of a specified process or outcome.

Innovation: A process of guided discovery and design.

Integration: A meshing of activities and practices oftentimes involving a health plan, a hospital, doctors, and diversified service into a unified closely working product or service. Integration is the link between processes, policies, and incentives to the actual delivery of clinical care at the patient level to improve patient health and deliver clinical excellence.

Key customer requirement: High-priority characteristics of current or future services and products that are described by customers, have actionable features, and where possible, include desired performance levels.

Key function: An organizational function believed, on the basis of evidence or expert consensus, to increase the probability of desired patient outcomes.

Key performance indicator: A process or result measure that reflects an important aspect of the overall performance of one or more business units.

Key process: A process believed, on the basis of evidence or expert consensus, to increase the probability of desired patient outcomes.

Knowledge: The capacity for effective action. It is the embodiment of what is learned.

Leader: A person in a position of authority over process(es), creating shared vision, seeking new ideas, creating meaning, demonstrating faith and courage, and establishing trust and accountability for improvement and change.

Leadership: The ability to build competence, creativity, and commitment through purpose, inspiration, demonstration of courage and faith, and modeling the way. Leadership is making dreams come true by activating the energy of others to nourish a collective vision with the necessary concentration and faith. *Source: Dick Richards.*

Learning: The enhancement of knowledge. It requires a will and skill.

Market-driven: We are responsive to customer requirements and perceptions that are articulated, and we meet those expectations. At the same time, we work with our customers to discover and design the capability to meet unarticulated needs. Finally, we strive to excel in customer knowledge. We bring the customer inside our organization to uncover and understand unexpressed needs and develop qualities in product and service that delight the customer.

Medical trend: The year-to-year increase or inflation in medical costs.

Operations: What is happening now and why.

Outcome criteria: Elements for evaluating end results in terms of health and satisfaction.

Pathway: Pathways are concurrent, multidisciplinary shorthand process tools for the complex coordinating and sequencing of health care interventions. They acknowledge key events that must occur within designated units of time and provide a base to predict the direction and movement of care toward outcomes. They improve efficiency and effectiveness of care through elimination of unnecessary variation in care processes.

Performance measurement: A systematic process for assessing what an organization does and achieves across multiple dimensions (for example, clinical, administrative, financial).

Planning: An element of the Allina culture that allows Allina to carry an idea through its development stages, ultimately leading to the idea's implementation. The process begins and ends with the customer.

Practice improvement: Although controlled clinical studies are the gold standard, they are not always feasible or affordable in practice. Outcome management is a structured alternative with statistical validity to related interventions to outcomes of routine care. This can validate or improve recognized practice.
Source: Intermountain Health Care.

Practice profiling: Assessment of patterns of health care service delivery and/or consumption over time; units of analysis could include individual physicians, groups of providers by specialty, department or clinic and defined populations.

Process: A goal-directed series of actions, events, mechanisms, or steps. A sequence of business activities that achieves a business result (creates value) for a customer.

Protocol: The plan or outline of a scientific experiment, treatment, or study.
Source: Office of Technology Report & Assessment, U.S. Congress, 1994.

Re-engineering: The fundamental rethinking and radical redesign of business processes or an entire business system to achieve dramatic improvements in critical measures of performance (for example, cost, quality, service, speed, capital).

Region: A reference to the entire territory served by Allina, currently including the greater metropolitan area of Minneapolis/St. Paul, Minnesota, eastern North Dakota, South Dakota, and western Wisconsin.

Regional: Regional is a subset of the Allina region and is an operational term used to define activities outside of the greater metropolitan area.

Respect and caring: The degree to which a patient, or designee, is involved in his or her own care decisions, and that those providing the services do so with sensitivity and respect for his or her needs and expectations and individual differences.

Safety: The degree to which the risk of an intervention and the risk in the care environment are reduced for the patient and others, including the health care provider.

Stakeholders: Parties who, by virtue of their roles and relationships with Allina, strongly impact our capacity to serve our customers and realize our vision (this includes employees, physicians, community leaders, suppliers, and regulators).

Standards: Standards are professionally developed expressions of the range of acceptable variation from a norm or criterion.

Systems: Language for telling the story about what is happening.

Team learning: The capacity to come together and bring all qualities of intelligence to contribute to the purpose.

Timeliness: The degree to which the care/intervention is provided to the patient at the time it is most beneficial or necessary.

Vision: Hopes for the future.

11

Instilling Pride, Joy, and Meaning in the Work of Health Care

F ew people in the health care industry speak about quality with the intensity and passion of Dr. Donald Berwick, President of the Institute of Health Improvement. To frame this chapter, the following is reprinted from the *New England Journal of Medicine*.[1]

Imagine two assembly lines, monitored by two foremen.

Foreman 1 walks the line, watching carefully. "I can see you all," he warns. "I have the means to measure your work, and I will do so. I will find those among you who are unprepared or unwilling to do your jobs, and when I do there will be consequences. There are many workers available for these jobs, and you can be replaced."

Foreman 2 walks a different line, and he too watches. "I am here to help you if I can," he says. "We are in this together for the long haul. You and I have a common interest in a job well done. I know that most of you are trying very hard, but sometimes things can go wrong. My job is to notice opportunities for improvement—skills that could be shared, lessons from the past, or experiments to try together—and to give you the means to do your work even better than you do now. I want to help the average ones among you, not just the exceptional few at either end of the spectrum of competence."

Which line works better? Which is more likely to do the job well in the long run? Where would you rather work?

In modern American health care, there are two approaches to the problem of improving quality—two theories of quality that describe the climate in which care is delivered. One will serve us well; the other probably will not.

The theory used by Foreman 1 relies on inspection to improve quality. We may call it the Theory of Bad Apples because those who subscribe to it believe that quality is best achieved by discovering bad apples and removing them from the lot. The experts call this mode "quality by inspection," and in the thinking of activists for quality in health care, it predominates under the guise of buying right, recertification, or deterrence through litigation. Such an outlook implies or establishes thresholds for acceptability, just as the inspector at the end of an assembly line decides whether to accept or reject finished goods. Those in health care who espouse the Theory of Bad Apples are looking hard for better tools of inspection. Such tools must have excellent measuring ability—high sensitivity and specificity, simultaneously—lest the malefactors escape or the innocent be made victims. They search for outlier—statistics far enough from the average that chance alone is unlikely to provide a good excuse. Bad Apples theorists publish mortality data, invest heavily in systems of case-mix adjustment, and fund vigilant regulators. Some measure their success by counting heads on platters.

The Theory of Bad Apples gives rise readily to what can be called the my-apple-is-just-fine-thank-you response on the part of the workers supervised by Foreman 1. The foreman has defined the rules of a game called "Prove you are acceptable," and that is what the workers play. The game is not fun, of course; the workers are afraid, angry, and sullen, but they play nonetheless. When quality is pursued in the form of a search for deficient people, those being surveyed play defense. They commonly use three tactics: kill the messenger (the foreman is not their friend, and the inspector even less so); distort the data or change the measurements (when possible, take control of the mechanisms that may do you harm); and if all else fails, turn somebody else in (and divert the foreman's attention).

Any good foreman knows how clever a frightened workforce can be. In fact, practically no system of measurement, at least none that measures people's performance, is robust enough to survive the fear of those who are measured. Most measurement tools eventually come under the control of those studied, and in their fear, such people do not ask what measurement can tell them, but rather how they can make it safe. The inspector says, "I will find you out if you are deficient." The subject replies, "I will therefore prove I am not deficient"—and seeks not understanding, but escape.

This game is played out repeatedly in health care. The view of a bad apple responsible for problems of quality shuts down the whole environment for inquiry, truth telling, learning, and improvement. It undermines the very soul of an organization—the meaning, pride, and joy in work—in which people are working hard and trying to do the right thing. An environment of quality engages those doing the work and focuses on process, learning, and overall improvement. Every defect is a treasure in this environment because in the discovery of defect and waste lies the chance for improvement. The Japanese call this Kaizen—the continuous search for processes to get better.[2]

Quality must be built and nurtured, not only in the formal structures and procedures of the organization, but in the people. It is in the people that the soul—the meaning and energy—of the organization resides.

This final chapter focuses the reader in a broad direction. It poses thoughts on how to drive out the fear in the environment and how to engage the soul of the organization in creating a different future that can instill joy, pride, and meaning in work within an environment of constant learning.

HISTORICAL PERSPECTIVE

Health care was among the first service industries to divide work tasks according to the factory model.[3] Hospitals were turned into factory-like organizations that delivered care to the sick. Specialties and subspecialties developed, and a hierarchical chain of command was installed. Care and service previously provided in homes and in the community were moved into the factory's organizations and further away from customers. The caregivers at the front line caring for patients executed orders and carried out procedures, often in fragmentation. An imbalance of power resulted as the tasks of nurses and other professionals were sharply divided from the tasks of physicians. Spiraling technology made the practice of health care even more industrialized. Customers became more objectified as body parts were treated and cared for, often in isolation of the whole person. The structure of the organization was adapted to serve needs of providers. Hierarchies emerged and the business of operating the organization and the activities of providing care and service in the organization became artificially separated.

CURRENT STATE OF HEALTH CARE

Health care is a big and costly industry. The financing and delivery of health care is increasingly complex. The purchasers and consumers of health care are letting it be known that trust in the health care system is eroding. For many who work in health care, it is an anxious time, characterized by increased pressure to demonstrate quality and value; reduce costs; and provide consumers with more time, information, participation, and choice in decisions affecting their health care. With alarming messages in the media about the health care industry, many who work in health care are struggling between two worlds—that of the inspired meaning and purpose derived from a profession that does good for humanity and that of dismay in the face of societal and business demands that say doing good is not enough.

The theme, "I love my work. I hate my job," resounds throughout the industry. In the turbulence of mergers, downsizing, inspection, and regulation, there is a call for leadership, creativity, and improvement. Physicians, nurses, managers, and employees, in partnership with the consumer, are increasingly challenged to have the knowledge and skills to redesign improved care processes, improve health, and reduce the burden of illness that society labors under today.

CHANGES SIGNALING A NEW FUTURE

Dr. Mitchell Rabkin, President and CEO, and Joyce Clifford, Vice-President of Nursing and Nurse-in-Chief, both at Beth Israel Hospital in Boston, are examples of leaders in health care today who have transformed a hierarchy into the inclusion of all health professionals, working in teams, to directly serve the customer.[4] The resources of the organization are focused to support them. Rabkin and Clifford created shared vision and focused the energy of the organization to create a new and better way of working. They developed systems to link providers directly to patient care. To examine a case study of the work at Beth Israel, consult *Web of Inclusion*, by Sally Helgesen.

Rabkin and Clifford tapped into the soul of their organization where pride, meaning, and joy in work reside. They used this energy to enable what Dick Richards refers to as artful work.[5] Together, they created a delivery system that restored dignity and power to those serving patients at the front line. They made training and development for people in the organization part of the process. And, most important, they recognized the patient and family as the center of all work.

It is an example of front-line empowerment. Beth Israel essentially returned to its roots, focusing on the patient and the close relationship with the community it was originally built to serve. A system of care—primary nursing—was implemented and later evolved into an integrated Clinical Practice Program. The hospital returned the work of care to a specified nurse-physician partnership and a care team that cares for a specific, individual patient, rather than individuals performing isolated tasks for many patients. Decision making was at the bedside, and systems for communication and continuity were established. The system increased each caregiver's knowledge and gave control of the process to the care team. This was artful work. Relationship, inquiry, learning, and pride replaced routinized execution of tasks. Knowledge at the front line was not limited to the customers' needs, but rather was extended to incorporate organizational goals and issues, including financial status. Information at the front line enables people to engage and contribute in the organization's progress. These changes have enabled the study of work process and outcomes, and improvement has flourished.

NEW PERSPECTIVE OF THE ORGANIZATION

Instead of thinking of the organization as a factory, think of it as an organism, consisting of relationships filled with meaning and potential, all linked in some way. The substance of the organization is the energy of people, and most work involves the interaction between people. Work is an essential channel of energy. Fragmentation, isolation, and lack of shared meaning and vision dissipate energy. Rabkin and Clifford knew this when they scanned the environment of Beth Israel in the early 1970s. Leaders can use people's energy to create, just as a potter uses clay, a painter applies pigment, or a poet uses words to convey images.[6] When thinking about this energy as the organization, the implications for leaders become clear.

Return to Artful Work

Before the era of mass production, people worked to create products of art and utility. They owned their work, and their work was an expression of themselves. Its accomplishment brought meaning, pride, and joy. The era of mass production removed people from their art as they moved into "jobs." Jobs robbed art and creativity from work as people produced fragmented units of a work product. This had the following four results[7]:

1. People began to see some things as artful and others as useful.
2. Work became something to do to achieve and survive, while art became viewed as leisure.

3. Rewards for work became more extrinsic.
4. Pride, joy, and meaning became lost.

People who study the nature of work and the creative process conclude that all work can be artful and all work can produce a sense of pride and joy. Some conditions are conducive to the creation of artful work. The following conditions are relevant to the subject of quality and the environment in which quality work can best be done:

- The reward for artful work is in the doing.
- The ambition of artful work is joy.
- Artful work demands that the artist own the work process.
- Artful work requires consistent and conscious use of the self.
- As the artist creates the work, the work creates the artist, and a cycle of development occurs.

If organizations are viewed from an industrial model, in which tasks are performed in a linear fashion, management approaches to organizations tend to focus on restructuring, using new technology, and moving people around. If organizations are viewed as being made up of people with the energy to do work that brings meaning, then management will focus on shared vision and values, commitment, and service—the lifeblood of pride, joy, and artful work.

Until people are engaged in a meaningful way with the work needed to achieve an organization's goals and vision, goals will remain unfulfilled and techniques will fail. Organizations that have leaders who create and inspire shared vision, who connect the work to the customer, and who actively engage the people doing the work in understanding and improving it, are those that will succeed. Quality organizations recognize and invest in the people that comprise the organization and seek their contributions.

Bring Out the Soul of an Organization

This soul, the seat of pride, joy, and meaning, lives underground in organizations, yet it is where the creative energy and force for positive change reside. People generally come to work to do a good job. This is exactly the energy that needs to be understood, nurtured, and embraced to build a culture of quality. A culture of quality calls for commitment, energy, creativity, and discipline to help people build new and better ways to get work done and serve customers.

Bringing out the soul of an organization requires organizations and the people in them to manage and work together. This new work calls on leaders and those on the front line. The leader will be asked to look at the ecology of the organization, the environment that allows people to grow, be excited and proud of their work, and connect their work with others. This means the dissolution of old boundaries, the release of paternalism or maternalism, and the start of work as adults, each responsible for his or her work, to each other and to the customer.

Engaging the soul of the organization requires humility. Speaking on the subject of artful work, one scientist said he became open to new possibilities when he realized that "he was a human being working with the scientific process rather than a scientist."[8] He noted that cultivating his own discipline with arrogance and bias separated him from what he could learn and create with others. To find the soul of the organization, the organization's members must see and seek other points of view, become clear about reality, test individual perceptions, and stay close to the customer to understand what they need and prefer. This is not an expert model, which assumes the expert knows best; this is a model of learning.

Move from Task to Commitment

Figure 11-1 shows a matrix that describes physician, employee, and management involvement.[9] The horizontal axis depicts a range from low to high of the quality of the relationship. The vertical axis depicts a range from low to high on ability to execute strategy. This matrix suggests that the greater the investment in the quality of the workforce, the level of physician engagement, and the relationships with all stakeholders (physicians, employees, and managers), the greater the ability to execute strategy. The upper right quadrant represents a partnership of shared vision, commitment, and aligned action. It implies the existence of a human resource environment that supports this partnership, incentives, development opportunities, career renewal strategies, and labor-management cooperation. The lower left quadrant represents an armed truce in which there is low trust, low involvement, and poor relationship quality. This is an environment of compliance, not commitment; an environment that is ill-equipped and insufficient to execute strategy, meet customer requirements, or learn and improve.

Develop a New Contract for Relationships

Moving to the level of involvement means being willing to fully engage and enter into a relationship. It requires that those involved ask themselves the following questions:[10]

FIGURE 11-1. Continuum of Physician-Employee-Management Involvement

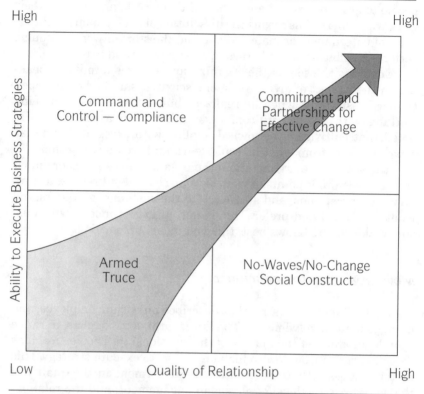

Reprinted, with permission, from Allina Health System, Minnetonka, Minn., 1998.

- Am I committed to the meaning of the work?
- Am I tenacious enough to do the work well?
- Do I care about the work itself?
- Can I express myself through the work?

The answers to these questions reflect some of the essential requirements of this relationship: commitment, tenacity, care and reflection, and self-expression.

Commitment   To engage also means choosing to commit to something. Compliance, mere going through the motions, cannot produce the pride, joy, and meaning that comes from commitment in the workplace. Commitment cannot be controlled or directed. People own their souls and energy and give them only by choice. Commitment must be inspired and earned.

Tenacity   Once committed, meaningful work requires people to be tenacious and dedicated and to apply themselves to the creation of the product. This means understanding vision in very practical terms and understanding the relationships required to achieve it and the effects of changing those relationships. The energy must be focused on what needs to be done and not on the distraction of the moment.

Commitment to meaningful work requires all the practice and discipline needed for the arts to work through the uncertainties and self doubts, to learn all there is to know about the craft and to practice it constantly. It requires a disciplined and informed approach to work. This means taking action, to do and perform the necessary functions. It means allocating time and energy to the performance of the work.

Care and Reflection   Commitment means believing in something enough to want it to happen. It requires stepping back to review and reflect on what has happened and how it happened so that knowledge and prediction can be applied to future work.

Self-Expression   As artists have long known, artful work is as much in the process as in its product. And working artfully requires ownership of the process. This ownership does not imply freedom from constraint, but joy in the process that advances work. Artists adhere to constraints. The painter works within the limits of canvas, photographers know the limits imposed by light and film, and potters know what they can and cannot do with the properties of clay. Yet with a well-designed and well-executed process, they are capable of extraordinary products.

Create a Shared Vision

It is exciting when people realize that they can create their future. Leading and working in an environment of shared vision requires new skills. Instead of controlling, motivating, and evaluating people, the leader has to listen to people and channel the energy of the people without diminishing it. Shared vision is required for collective commitment and aligned action. Through the process of creating shared vision, the people of the organization align energy and bring vision into reality. To commit to quality means moving from one model that all knowledge resides in the head of people at the top of the organization to another in which knowledge is placed in the hands of people throughout the organization.

As Peter Drucker has observed, another phenomena is occurring: "In new information-based organizations that are presently evolving, knowledge and expertise will be predominantly distributed at the bottom, held by those with the most direct contact with the customer."[11] In today's successful organizations, managers are becoming increasingly dependent on employees for knowledge.

WHAT WOULD AN ARTFUL ORGANIZATION LOOK LIKE?[12]

In an organization in which work would once again combine utility and art, a number of factors would exist: All forms of human energy would be welcomed, validated, and viewed as a contribution to the organization. Joy would be intrinsic to the work processes. People would be involved in work that is congruent with the requirements of their spirits and souls. It would have meaning. Commitment would be the norm. People would manage their own processes and have the necessary resources to do so.

In an organization that seeks to combine utility and art, communication that is authentic and actively encouraged would be common. People would be engaged with and committed to the organization's purpose, and the processes, products, and methods they used would always be in service to that purpose. In that way, all aspects of work would have meaning. Decisions would be logical, meaningful, and relevant.

The Leader's Work in an Artful Organization

In organizations in which the soul has been brought to life, leaders have new roles and responsibilities. Leaders must be experts in communicating the purpose and meaning of work and concentrating the energy of others through providing focus. They also provide faith—the belief in something that cannot be proven. Organizational crises are often related to faith. We simply do not trust ourselves and each other. At some point, a crisis of confidence may occur when employees wonder, can we really do this? In this situation, leaders must have an internal gauge and trust it. They must be experts in developing faith in the vision, in themselves, and in others in the organization.

The leader in quality uses the energy of the people in the organization to build success, just as the painter uses the energy of paint and the poet uses the energy of words. The leader must be acquainted with the qualities of human energy, as the painter understands the color spectrum. Leaders must speak from their souls with personal purpose and confidence.

Implications for Leaders of Developing a Quality Organization

Leaders who develop a quality organization rely on the following five fundamental tenets:[13]

1. Challenge the process.
2. Inspire shared vision.
3. Enable others to act.
4. Model the way.
5. Encourage the heart.

These tenets are shown in figure 11-2 with what Kouzes and Posner call the Ten Commitments of Leadership.

Challenge the Process In their research, Kouzes and Posner found that the leader's primary contribution is to recognize good ideas, support them, and challenge the system to get new and better ways adopted. In the book *Diffusion of Innovation*, these leaders are called the early adopters of innovation.[14] They know the risks, but they proceed anyway. In short, they lead. Warren Bennis, professor and student of leadership, characterized these leaders as learners. They learn by leading and often learn best by leading in the face of obstacles, when they are committed to review and reflect on their experience.[15]

Inspire a Shared Vision Leaders have dreams of what could be and confidence in their ability to make extraordinary results happen. The leader shares this vision and is able to communicate in a way that inspires commitment—vividly, enthusiastically, passionately. The leader knows the people in the organization—their hopes, dreams, personal visions, beliefs—and can connect to the people authentically in a way that strengthens the purpose. The leader uses dialogue, not monologue, and actively engages others so that they can create the future together.

FIGURE 11-2. Ten Commitments of Leadership

Practices	Commitments
Challenging the Process	1. **Search out** challenging opportunities to change, grow, innovative, and improve.
	2. **Experiment,** take risks, and learn from the accompanying mistakes.
Inspiring a Shared Vision	3. **Envision** an uplifting and ennobling future.
	4. **Enlist** others in a common vision by appealing to their values, interests, hopes, and dreams.
Enabling Others to Act	5. **Foster** collaboration by promoting cooperative goals and building trust.
	6. **Strengthen** people by giving power away, providing choice, developing competence, assigning critical tasks, and offering visible support.
Modeling the Way	7. **Set** the example by behaving in ways that are consistent with shared values.
	8. **Achieve** small wins that promote consistent progress and build commitment.
Encouraging the Heart	9. **Recognize** individual contributions to the success of every project.
	10. **Celebrate** team accomplishments regularly.

Reprinted, with permission, from J. M. Kouzes and B. Z. Posner, *The Leadership Challenge* (San Francisco: Jossey-Bass, 1995).

Enable Others to Act   Leaders use the word *we*. They have humility, enlist assistance, and believe in teamwork. They engage the people who must live with a project's results. They create an environment of ownership and confidence. They give away power—ensuring that people have the information, tools, and authority to do their work. The leader also creates a safe environment to take risks. They build trust through consistent trustworthy actions. They look for overall improvement in processes, not bad apples.

Model the Way   Leaders never ask anyone to do anything they would be unwilling to do themselves. They set example through daily acts. Their principles and values are embodied by what they do. They need to put things into operation by measuring performance, meeting schedules and budgets, evaluating performance, giving feedback, constantly improving their methods, and doing the concrete work of the organization. Failure to do so erodes employees' faith that the vision can become reality. People need to see, step-by-step, that effective action can be and is taken to produce results. Vision without clear strategy and action becomes just a grand fable rather than a call to action.

Encourage the Heart   Leaders instill and keep the faith, the belief that success will be achieved. They celebrate the gains that have been made, and in doing so, encourage the self-esteem and pride of accomplishment in others. Leaders help reconcile the science and the soul of the organization. They bring together the most exacting, rigorous data and logic with the search for meaning, the passion, sheer joy, and pride in doing work well. They concentrate the energy and faith of the people to create.

A BALANCE OF SCIENCE AND SOUL: AN EXAMPLE

Dr. Jim Ehlen, President of Allina Health System, has a story that embodies the balance of science and soul. It is a story about Michael, a fourth-grade student who has asthma. Michael's claims history showed a pattern of acute exacerbations and emergency care and the absence of any ongoing primary care relationship. This child was not receiving optimal care. He might have been labeled noncompliant, his family labeled uninvolved, and the case lost to the health care system. Decades ago, Michael might have had a family doctor or neighborhood nurse who knew all about him and his family and did whatever it took to keep him well. Today it is harder. People move and change health plans. People access care at many sites, and information is often fragmented. What precisely constitutes optimal care continues to be defined, and it is difficult for clinicians to always be current in what is better practice. Providing health care carries an obligation to care for people like Michael. Dr. Ehlen underscores this obligation:[16]

Today, it's tough for any one physician to keep track of everything that's happening to a patient. But at Allina, we still believe it's possible to provide the kind of care and oversight people used to get from their neighborhood or country doctor. We're not one doctor, but we are one system. Because we have access to all the pieces along the way, from health plan to clinic to hospital, we have the ability to manage the clinical care and service every step of the way.

It is not going to be easy. We will go slowly, incrementally, asking the right questions and reaffirming our work as we move ahead. We will measure care and service improvement and share the results. Then we'll try to improve some more.

How will we know if we have succeeded? Well, the quality improvement process never ends, but I, for one, will consider it a major success if we can learn from Michael about how to best work with him and his family. If Michael can get his asthma controlled because we have done our jobs of providing the information, clinical care, and service he and his family need to achieve the best possible health, that's success.

This measure of success comes from the president of one of the nation's largest health care systems. Size, in this corporation, is an opportunity—an opportunity to design models that improve health across a continuum of need, choice, providers, and services. Information and improvement serve as integrating features. So does science—evidence-based best practice guidelines, measurement and improvement methods, change theory and its strategies. There is also soul, the work of health care serves people and improves their health. Asthma care has a human face, like Michael and his unique needs and circumstances.

PRESENT STATE OF QUALITY

Variance regarding quality and the implementation of quality systems in the health care industry is still great. The emphasis here is the word *system*. Millions of examples of quality improvement initiatives focus on specific topics. That's a start. Exemplars of empowered environments in which leaders are committed to people having information and owning their work process do exist. That's a start. Leaders and spokespersons in health care espouse quality and improvement. That, too, is a start.

This book is suggesting more. It is calling for a systematic integrated approach to evaluation and improvement across the organization. It calls for examining best-in-class results and using the available science and tools with the same rigor and passion with which the industry approaches new cures.

Quality is not easy work. It requires science, discipline, and constant practice. It also requires soul—the courage to face reality, a passion to see a better future, and the tenacity to do what it takes. It recognizes the energy of those who give and receive health care. Everyone involved wants the process, the experience, and result to meet customers' needs. Health care is in a broken and fragmented system. The President's Commission on Consumer Protection and its recent publication of a Consumer Bill of Rights attest to the point that all is not well. What is not well involves individuals and the systems in which they work.

Quality is critical work, whether the activity is at a level of an individual health plan member's question or the redesign of a large system. We are all in this together, and we all need to develop the following fundamental qualities:

- Seeing health care as a whole system, requiring understanding and managing
- Having the curiosity to understand and predict change and to look for new ways through experimentation and testing
- Being committed and informed board members and leaders who move from theory to action by declaring quality as a business imperative, defining strategies to integrate quality into all aspects of the organization, and rigorously measuring process and results for evidence of improvement
- Creating work environments that engage and invest in the people doing the work, inspiring the soul, and ensuring the science and technique (This includes developing shared vision and values, commitment, competency and the endurance to stick with it. It also requires tools and methods to systematically and continuously measure the perspective of physicians and employees around dimensions of pride, joy, and meaning, and taking action on what is discovered.)
- Involving customers in the design and delivery of services, products, and processes based on their needs and preferences
- Developing the skills, technologies, and decision-support tools that engage customers in decisions about choices in lifestyle, treatment, and care options
- Using a systematic approach to managing information and improving its use
- Knowing and responding to the most serious defects and most promising opportunities in the system

- Working to restore the faith and trust of the public in health care by making safety an explicit agenda, engaging in open dialogue with consumers, and admitting to error and needed improvements when they are identified
- Visibly celebrating gains and innovations that better serve the customer

CONCLUSION

Inside each health care organization and within the nation's health care system as a whole, quality must increasingly have a visible, tangible, and intentional role. This work does not have to be done in isolation. The pursuit of excellence in serving customers has its own gravitational pull. People will engage in the effort when it is clear to them what the effort is. There are significant resources, including the National Foundation for Patient Safety, the Malcolm Baldrige National Award Program through the National Institute of Standards and Technology, the American Society of Quality Control, Agency for Health Care Policy and Research, the Juran Institute, the Institute for Health Improvement, the Picker Institute, the Healthcare Forum, accrediting bodies such as the Joint Commission on Accreditation of Healthcare Organizations and the National Committee on Quality Assurance, professional medical and nursing associations, and associations such as the American Hospital Association, the Voluntary Hospitals of America, to name a few. Each have specific expertise, from reducing error, understanding customer value points, and building leadership and organizational capacity in quality to examining variation, evaluating what constitutes the right care, and understanding end-of-life care.

With the information, tools, and authority in the hands of people who directly serve the customer, what is the unique role of leaders? It resides in being familiar with the people who, collectively, are the soul of our organizations. With the crisis of confidence about health care and the turbulent changes confronting the system, people are struggling to find a future worthy of their past. The emphasis in this book has been on how leaders can engender belief from their followers. In quality, leaders must also believe in their followers and have faith in all human possibilities. Leaders, through their own insatiable curiosity, can reawaken that natural curiosity in people. At their core, those who work in health care are learners and action-takers. Kotter best describes the habits of such learners and action-takers as follows: risk-taking or the willingness to push oneself out of comfort zones, the practice of humble and honest self-reflection, the aggressive collection of opinions and ideas from others, the skill of careful listening to others, and the willingness to view life with an open mind.[17]

Reconnecting to the soul—to the meaning, pride, and joy in work—creates energy. This reconnection will create the energy for followers to become leaders, for leaders to become followers, for them to become equals, walking a common path with one, common customer. As Warren Bennis says, "None of us is as smart as all of us."[18]

References

1. Berwick, D., "Continuous Quality Improvement as an Ideal in Health Care," Sounding Board, *New England Journal of Medicine* 320(1) (Jan. 5, 1989): 53–6.

2. Imai, M., *The Key to Japanese Competitive Success* (New York: Random House, 1986).

3. Helgesen, S., *The Web of Inclusion* (New York: Doubleday, 1995): 129.

4. Helgesen, pp. 125–63.

5. Richards, D., *Artful Work: Awakening Joy, Meaning, and Commitment in the Workplace* (San Francisco: Berrett-Koehler, 1995).

6. Richards, p. 6.

7. Richards, p. 8.

8. Whyte, D., author of *The Heart Aroused*, speaking at Bretton Woods Gathering of Practitioners in Learning Organizations, 1994.

9. Howe, M., and J. Morath, *Employee-Management Involvement Model* (HealthSpan, Minneapolis, Minn., 1995).

10. Richards, p. 30.

11. Hesselbein, F., M. Goldsmith, and R. Beckhard (eds), *The Leader of the Future: New Visions, Strategies, and Practices for the Next Era* (San Francisco, Jossey-Bass, 1996).

12. Richards, pp. 95–104.

13. Kouzes, J. M., and B. Z. Posner, *The Leadership Challenge, How to Keep Getting Extraordinary Things Done in Organizations* (San Francisco: Jossey-Bass, 1995): 18.

14. Rogers, E. M., *Diffusion of Innovation*, 4th edition (New York: The Free Press, 1995): 252–80.

15. Bennis, W., and P. W. Biederman, *Organizing Genius: The Secrets of Creative Collaboration* (Reading, Mass.: Addison-Wesley, 1997): 1.

16. Ehlen, J. K., President, Allina Health Systems, Minnetonka, Minn. Prepared remarks for the Allina Leadership on Vision and Quality, 1998.

17. Kotler, J., *Leading Change* (Boston: Harvard Business School Press, 1996): 183.

18. Bennis, p. 1.

Suggested Readings

Blanchard, K., and M. O'Connor, *Managing by Values* (San Francisco: Berrett-Koehler, 1997).

Block, P., *Choosing Service over Self-Interest* (San Francisco: Berrett-Koehler, 1993).

Bluestone, B., and I. Bluestone, *Negotiating the Future: A Labor Perspective on American Business* (New York: BasicBooks, Division of HarperCollins, 1992).

Chaleff, I., *The Courageous Follower* (San Francisco: Berrett-Koehler, 1995).

Chawla, S., and J. Renesch, *Learning Organizations* (Portland, Ore.: Productivity Press, 1995).

Davenport, T. H., *Information Ecology: Mastering the Information and Knowledge Environment* (New York: Oxford University Press, 1997).

DePree, M., *Leadership Is an Art* (New York: Dell, 1989).

Friedman, E., *The Right Thing* (San Francisco: Jossey-Bass, 1996).

Gubman, E. L., *Talent Solution: Aligning Strategy and People to Achieve Extraordinary Results* (New York: McGraw-Hill, 1998).

Handy, C., *The Age of Paradox* (Cambridge, Mass.: Harvard Business School Press, 1994).

Katzenbach, J. R., and D. Smith, *The Wisdom of Teams: Creating the High Performance Organization* (Boston: Harvard Business School Press, 1993).

Kouzes, J. M., and Posner, B. Z., *The Leadership Challenge* (San Francisco: Jossey-Bass, 1987).

Peck, M. S., *The Different Drum: Community Making and Peace* (New York: Touchstone, 1987).

Ryback, D., *Putting Emotional Intelligence to Work: Successful Leadership Is More Than IQ* (Boston: Butterworth-Heinemann, 1998).

Stewart, T., *Intellectual Capital: The New Wealth of Organizations* (New York: Currency/Doubleday, 1997).

Whyte, D., *The Heart Aroused: Poetry and the Preservation of the Soul in Corporate America* (New York: Doubleday, 1994).

Worthley, J. A., *The Ethics of the Ordinary in Healthcare* (Chicago: Health Administration Press, 1997).

Index

243